SOCIETY FOR NEW TESTAMENT STUDIES

MONOGRAPH SERIES

General Editor: G. N. Stanton

55

MEDICINE, MIRACLE AND MAGIC IN
NEW TESTAMENT TIMES

Medicine, Miracle and Magic in New Testament Times

HOWARD CLARK KEE

William Goodwin Aurelio Professor of Biblical Studies
Boston University

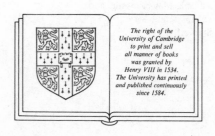

The right of the
University of Cambridge
to print and sell
all manner of books
was granted by
Henry VIII in 1534.
The University has printed
and published continuously
since 1584.

CAMBRIDGE UNIVERSITY PRESS

CAMBRIDGE
LONDON   NEW YORK   NEW ROCHELLE
MELBOURNE   SYDNEY

Published by the Press Syndicate of the University of Cambridge
The Pitt Building, Trumpington Street, Cambridge CB2 1RP
32 East 57th Street, New York, NY 10022, USA
10 Stamford Road, Oakleigh, Melbourne 3166, Australia

First published 1986

Printed in Great Britain at
the University Press, Cambridge

British Library cataloguing in publication data

Kee, Howard Clark
Medicine, miracle and magic in New Testament times −
(Society for New Testament Studies; 55)
1. Bible. N.T. − Criticism,
interpretation, etc.   2. Miracles.
3. Healing in the Bible
I. Title.   II. Series
226'.7   BS2545.H4

Library of Congress cataloguing in publication data

Kee, Howard Clark.
Medicine, miracle and magic in New Testament
times.
(Monograph series / Society for New Testament
Studies; 55)
Bibliography.
Includes indexes.
1. Medicine in the Bible.   2. Medicine, Greek and
Roman.   3. Miracles.   4. Medicine, Magic, mystic, and
spagiric.   I. Title.   II. Series: Monograph series
(Society for New Testament Studies); 55.
R135.5.K44   1986   220.8'61   85-31327

ISBN 0 521 32309 6

For JACOB NEUSNER
Esteemed Colleague and Friend

CONTENTS

PREFACE

After the completion of my study, *Miracle in the Early Christian World* (New Haven: Yale University Press, 1983), my continued interest in the phenomenon of healing in the New Testament led me to an investigation of another mode of healing from this period: medicine. It quickly became clear to me that this aspect of Graeco-Roman culture did not fall into a simple, neat category, but was as subject to change as I had discovered miracle to be. The result of these preliminary explorations was the determination to investigate in their inter-relationships to each other the three approaches to healing from this period: medicine, miracle and magic.

With the encouragement of my colleagues at Boston University, I applied for and was granted a Summer Stipend from the National Endowment for the Humanities. My research was carried out in the superbly equipped and staffed library of the Wellcome Institute of the History of Medicine in London in the summer of 1984. Conversations with colleagues at the Studiorum Novi Testamenti Societas at its annual meeting later that summer in Basel led me to undertake converting my research notes into a monograph on the subject. It was my hope that the assembling of this evidence and the analytical framework in which it was placed might help to enrich our understanding of the context in which the New Testament was written and in which the early Christian movement spread so rapidly.

The preparation of this monograph was aided by friends and colleagues here in the USA, and especially in Boston: the staffs of various libraries in the Boston area (Boston University School of Theology, the Boston Athenaeum, Boston College), colleagues at the New York New Testament Seminar, the staff of the Graduate Division of Religious Studies at Boston University. A special word of thanks is due to Professor James H. Charlesworth of Princeton Theological Seminary, who not only introduced me to the medical

MS from Qumran, but also prepared it for publication in the appendix to the present work.

HOWARD CLARK KEE
Boston University

INTRODUCTION
DEFINITIONS AND CONTEXTS FOR HEALING

In every age and in every social setting, a primary concern of human beings is health. This concern manifests itself in two distinct modes: (1) the eagerness to maintain the health of the body, and the negative corollary, which is the overcoming of sickness; (2) the basic human need to discern some framework of meaning by which the cause of sickness, suffering, and disability can be understood, and by which these universal experiences of frailty and vulnerability can be incorporated into a view of the world and humanity's place within it. The importance of these issues for the New Testament is broad and deep, as is apparent from the gospels, the Acts, and the various letters. Of the approximately 250 literary units into which the first three gospels are divided in a typical synopsis,[1] one fifth either describe or allude to the healing and exorcistic activities of Jesus and the disciples. Of the seven "signs"[2] reported in John to have been done by Jesus, four involve healing or restoration. Of the seventy literary units in John, twelve either describe his healing activity or refer to the signs which he performed.

Often overlooked is the importance Paul attached to healing. He lists healing and working miracles among the charismatic gifts (I Cor 12:9–10). Later in that chapter, where he is describing these gifts in order of importance, he ranks miracles and healings after the gift of teaching (I Cor 12:28–30). In II Cor 12:12, "signs, wonders and miracles" – which presumably include healings – are indicated as "the signs of the apostle" that have been performed among the Corinthian Christians. Far from viewing miracles as falsely prized by his opponents in Corinth,[3] Paul draws attention in Rom 15:19 to the power of signs and wonders which have been accomplished by him, through the Spirit, as divine confirmation of his ministry throughout the entire quadrant of the Mediterranean world, stretching from Jerusalem to the Adriatic.

This interpretation of "signs and wonders" is assumed by the author of Acts, who builds on the biblical phrase (2:19, quoting Joel 2:28–32), finding in the "mighty works and wonders and signs ... which God did through [Jesus] in your midst" (Acts 2:22) the divine attestation of Jesus as "Lord and Christ" (2:36). The signs and wonders attributed to the apostles throughout Acts (2:43; 5:12; 6:8; 7:36; 14:3; 15:12) are represented as divine confirmation of the apostolic undertaking and are specified in the apostolic prayer (4:30) as pre-eminently works of healing. Similarly in Hebrews, "signs, wonders and miracles" are described as confirmatory activity of the Holy Spririt in the midst of God's people (Heb 2:3–4). In James 5:13–16, the efficacy of prayer in accomplishing healing is asserted.

James mentions, however, that the prayer for healing is to be accompanied by an "anointing ... with oil" (5:14). Does this imply that the early church was combining simple medical technique with healing in response to prayer? Are we to see, as scholars have often suggested, a similar medical or even magical technique in Jesus' application of spittle to the tongue of the deaf-mute in Mk 7:33 and to the eyes of the blind man in Mk 8:23? Is Jesus adopting, or being conformed by the bearers of the tradition to patterns of miracle-working, or medicine, or magic that were alive in the world of the first century? Or, to phrase the question from another perspective, to what extent does the healing tradition of the New Testament display continuity with the biblical and post-exilic Jewish world view(s) on the subject? Or is the perception of healing in the New Testament and early Christian tradition largely derived from standard patterns in the Graeco-Roman world?

Before turning to an analysis of these healing traditions of Judaism and the late Hellenistic world, it may be useful to offer a preliminary discussion and definition of the three major modes of healing – medicine, miracle and magic – which are in competition with each other during this period. As we shall see, it is often the case that, in any given document or tradition, distinctions among them become blurred, but as heuristic devices it is essential to trace how each of these terms represents a significantly different approach to healing with regard to both the cause and the cure of human afflictions. In the main body of the present work, Chapter 1 focusses on the attitudes toward healing within Judaism in the biblical and post-biblical periods. Chapter 2 traces the development of medicine in the Greek and Roman worlds, with special attention to those phases contemporary with the New Testament. Chapter 3 discusses the phenomenon of miracle, and the reactions to it from the Roman world. The final chapter looks at magic, from the perspective of ancient evidence as well as from that of modern interpreters.

The modes of healing with which each of these chapters is concerned can be defined in ways which sharply differentiate each from the other. Yet historically, they occur in documents and contexts which imply the shading over from one category into another. Of great importance, furthermore, is to recognize that during the period of our inquiry – and perhaps at any time – none of these three strategies for dealing with the problems of sickness and health was a firmly fixed entity, but that instead each developed in distinctive ways under the influence of the changing social and cultural context. And even from one socio-cultural setting to another during any single epoch, there were significant variations which must be taken into account if faithful historical analysis and reconstruction are to be achieved. Convenient for the chronological and conceptual purposes of our inquiry are the towering medical figures who left an enduring impress on the history of medicine and health in the western world and whose lifetimes bracket the Graeco-Roman period: Hippocrates (460–350 B.C.) and Galen (130–200 A.D.). Hippocrates figured importantly in the period of classical Greek philosophy, as mention of him in the writings of Aristotle attests.[4] Galen represents himself as the recoverer of the Hippocratic tradition, and as such has had a dominant influence on the subsequent history of medicine, in both the medieval Arab world and in the post-medieval West.[5] Yet running concurrently with the medical tradition, at times in competition with it, and at other times overlapping with it, were the two other means of dealing with sickness and suffering: miracle and magic.

These three related sets of phenomena may be defined as follows. *Medicine* is a method of diagnosis of human ailments and prescription for them based on a combination of theory about and observation of the body, its functions and malfunctions. *Miracle* embodies the claim that healing can be accomplished through appeal to, and subsequent action by the gods, either directly or through a chosen intermediary agent. *Magic* is a technique, through word or act, by which a desired end is achieved, whether that end lies in the solution to the seeker's problem or in damage to the enemy who has caused the problem. Since each of these instruments of health presupposes a different theory of the cause of sickness or disability, it is essential to differentiate some of the ways in which sickness is understood as originating. These include the theory that human difficulties are the work of demons, for which exorcism is the appropriate cure; or that they are the results of a magical curse, for which counter-magic must be invoked; or that they are functional disorders of the body, which call for medical diagnosis and a prescribed remedy.

Complicating the picture of the various modes by which human health was sought in this period is a series of factors. In literature and documents from the Graeco-Roman period there is evidence of debates about whether or not the gods were involved in human healing, and if so, by what means. For example, Asklepios was viewed simultaneously as the patron of physicians and as the beneficent god who acted directly to heal suppliants. In addition, those who claimed to perform miracles were charged by their detractors with doing magic. And indeed, some features of miracle-working resemble the techniques of magicians, just as the magicians invoke the names of the miracle-working gods. In an older study of the relationship between medicine, magic and religion, W.H.R. Rivers, who discussed the inter-relation among these phenomena, observed that physicians, miracle workers and magicians may all seek to overcome a disease by abstracting some evil factor from the body, or by treating something which has been connected with the body (such as hair, sweat, excrement, or food). For us to differentiate among the modes requires, therefore, an exact knowledge, not only of the rites performed, but also of the presuppositions and assumptions about reality in general and the human condition in particular, in order to determine in which category the healing action falls.[6] If the technique is effective of itself in overcoming a hostile force, then the action is magical. If it is viewed as the intervention of the god or goddess, then it is miraculous. If it is a facilitating of the natural function of the body, then it is medical. In his introduction to Rivers' study, G.E. Smith observes with regard to healing in what we would call primitive societies:

> The fundamental aim of primitive religion was to safeguard life, which was achieved by certain simple mechanical procedures based upon rational inference, but often upon false premises. Primitive medicine sought to achieve the same end, and not unnaturally used the same means. Hence in the beginning religion and medicine were parts of the same discipline, of which magic was merely a department.

He continues this assessment with the observation that in some cultures the three factors are nearly indistinguishable, while in others, "the name of medicine can hardly be said to exist, so closely is man's attitude toward disease identical with that which he adopts toward other classes of natural phenomena". To differentiate a religious from a medical approach to healing, Smith observes, requires that one take carefully into account "a certain attitude toward the world".[7]

It would be a serious historical error to assume, however, that the medical approach to health was the province of the intellectuals, while religion and magic were left to the ignorant, or that intellectuals universally respected the medical profession and shared its basic outlook. Pliny the Elder, in his *Natural History*, in fact deplores the rise of the medical profession, which he regards as having come to Rome through an invasion of crafty, unscrupulous Greek charlatans. Instead of relying on the traditional natural remedies which he admires (XXIX.1), the so-called medical art has taken over, which is "lucrative beyond all the rest". These physicians have abandoned the substances which nature intended for healing and which are everywhere available at little or no cost, and instead insist on extremely costly medicaments from foreign lands, and require the services of their laboratories (*officines*). These highly popular and economically successful developments, Pliny declares, attest to "the fraudulent disposition of mankind, combined with an ingenuity prompted by lucre". These medical schemers promise everyone "an extension of life − that is, if he will pay for it". One of Pliny's chief candidates for medical charlatanry was the well-known Greek physician, Asclepiades, who turned to medicine after having failed to earn enough as a rhetorician. Developing his theories largely on the basis of conjectures, and tailoring his cures to suit the needs and comforts of his gullible clients, the latter enjoyed enormous popularity and financial success − all without training or experience in medicine. The chief factor in his success, Pliny asserts, is "the follies of magic" (XXVI.9). Pliny finds support for his point of view about medicine from Cato, whom he quotes concerning physicians:

> They are a most iniquitous and intractable race, and you may take my word as the word of a prophet, when I tell you that whenever that nation [= Greece] shall bestow its literature upon Rome it will mar everything; and that all the sooner if it sends its physicians among us. They have conspired among themselves to murder all barbarians with their medicine; a profession which they exercise for lucre, in order that they win our confidence, and dispatch us all the more easily. Have nothing to do with physicians![8]

Pliny's own approach to matters of health assumes that the basic principles of healing are ingredient in the natural order. Nature has seen to it that medicines are everywhere available, even in the desert, so that there are "at every point ... wonderful examples of that well-known sympathy and antipathy" (*Nat. Hist.* XXIV.1). We shall see that in medicine from the earliest time the principles of sympathetic and homeopathic treatment are basic for therapy. We might ask parenthetically whether these remedies represent medicine or magic. Pliny observes that for all forms of life and for every inanimate substance there is a pairing of opposites. These natural remedies have been "provided everywhere", cost nothing and are easily discovered – things that in fact are basic to the support of life (*Nat. Hist.* XXIV.1.4).

Later, Pliny continues, human deceit and profiteering led some men to set themselves forth as experts in these matters, but unlike those who shared folk remedies, these schemers charged fees for their services and prescribed costly remedies from distant lands, and did so for personal profit. The necessary medicaments "form the daily dinner of even the poorest" and could be found "in the kitchen garden" (XXVI.21.5). If only that fact were recognized, then "none of the arts would be cheaper than medicine". These medicaments are available throughout the natural world, even in animals (XXVIII.120). Why, then, have these universally available resources been neglected, replaced instead by the costly prescriptions of the professionals?

It is the fault of the medical profession itself. Those who pioneered in that profession attributed the origins of their art to the gods, especially to Asklepios, apparently to lend an aura of sanctity to their enterprise, even though legend reported that the god had been struck by lightning for bringing someone back to life (*Nat. Hist.* XXIX.1.3). At Cos, where there was a shrine to Asklepios that was visited by the ailing, who left behind testimonies to the healing powers of the god, the founder of the Greek medical tradition, Hippocrates, was born. Taking advantage of the burning of the Temple of Asklepios, Hippocrates had developed a medical clinic at Cos, which launched medicine as a revenue-producing enterprise. After sketching the leading figures and the various schools of thought which developed in the medical tradition after Hippocrates in Greece, Alexandria and Sicily, Pliny renews his attack on Asclepiades and his successors who made enormous fortunes as physicians to the emperors (XXIX.5.6–8). Pliny concedes that "with great distinction" Hippocrates had laid down rules for medical practice, including abundant advice about the use of herbs, but gradually this tradition, he charges, "degenerated into words and mere talk", with more interest in listening to lectures than in searching out medicinal plants (XXIV.6.11). It was in the late first century B.C. that Pliny's favourite medical villain, Asclepiades, had come from Bithynia to Rome (fl. 90–75 B.C.) and had taken the people of Rome by storm. Though he was a professor of rhetoric and wholly lacking in medical experience or knowledge of natural remedies, he had developed a theoretical system which, Pliny says, "brought round to his view almost the whole human race, just as if he had been ... an apostle from heaven" (XXVI.7.13). The five basic rules of his system are neither exceptional nor exceptionable: fasting from food, abstinence from wine, massage, walking, carriage-riding. In addition, his modes of therapy included rocking beds, baths of hot water and hot air. Pliny's chief objection to Asclepiades was that he was so powerfully influenced by "Magian deceits" that he destroyed confidence in all herbal remedies (XXVI.9.1).

The objections Pliny raised to magic are even stronger than those he made concerning medicine. He regarded magic as an exploitation of medicine, by which its practitioners claimed to "promote health ... under the guise of a higher and holier system". It was his opinion that magic had increased its appeal by adding both religion and astrology to its approach to human health. So great was the interest and so spread across the intellectual spectrum, he notes, that even philosophers such as Plato, Pythagoras, Empedocles and Democritus went overseas to learn it (XXX.2.9), just as it had influenced the Jews, such as Moses (XXX.2.11). It had spread throughout the western part of the empire, although it had originated in the East. It had become an obsession of even the emperor, Nero, whose "greatest wish was to command the gods". Pliny thought that the essentially fraudulent nature of magic was apparent in that even gullible Nero, after having devoted such enormous wealth and energy to its pursuit, eventually abandoned it (XXX.5.15). Yet even as Pliny was denouncing magic as "detestable, vain, and idle", he acknowledged that it had what might be called "shadows of the truth" (XXX.6.17). Revealing is the fact that when Pliny begins to describe the remedies prescribed by the magicians – which he does at great length – they are scarcely distinguishable from those that he represents elsewhere in *Natural History* as natural remedies. Indeed, he slips into such phrases when he is presenting the magician's cures as "I find that" and "very useful too" (XXX.10.30; 11.31). Even after characterizing the magicians as "fraudulent charlatans" (XX.8.27) in connection with their claims about the magical powers of the hyena, he reports that "a sure safeguard against miscarriage is an amulet of gazelle leather containing white flesh from a hyena's breast, seven hairs from a hyena and the genital organ of a stag" (XXVIII.27.98). Or again, he merely states without comment, pejorative or otherwise, that "the extreme end of the hyena's intestine prevails against the injustice of leaders and potentates, bringing success to petitions and a happy issue to trials and lawsuits, if it is merely kept on the person" (XXX.27.106). It is as though Pliny, having outwardly denounced magic, is unconsciously persuaded by the claims of its partisans.

Clearly for Pliny, and for others in the Roman world, as we shall see, the distinctions that they make between natural healing, medicine and magic have nothing to do with what might be styled in our modern era as rational cause-and-effect, to say nothing of so-called scientific objectivity. As we shall have occasion to note, modern historians of science have tried to read these distinctions back into the Hellenistic and Roman periods. The question is not whether hidden powers produce visible results. On that there would be wide agreement. The question for us to ask is: in what framework of meaning are these powers understood as being at work?

When we raise this kind of question, the issues surrounding health can perhaps be brought into focus through the posing of two further questions for which the various segments of the Graeco-Roman world gave decidedly different answers. (1) By what powers can human beings gain and retain good health? (2) To what extent is the human condition the result of inescapable factors constituted by nature itself, and to what extent can effective appeal for aid or access to power be made through superhuman agencies? As we have already observed, there were not simple answers to these questions during the major period of our interest – from the late Hellenistic period to the end of the second century and the close of the Antonine era. Our aim is to clarify the relationships among these three approaches to healing – medicine, miracle and magic – rather than to trace the history of any one of them in detail. In the process we shall examine the evidence from the centuries before and after the birth of Jesus in the context of the various socio-cultural settings in which the phenomena appear, bearing in mind the different assumptions about reality that are implicit in and expressed through the evidence.

Attitudes and praxes towards sickness among the rabbis, as well as in Greek and Roman writers, are compared with the Bible, especially the New Testament. Healing is pursued through: 1) medicine, physical (and occasionally) psychological observations and natural remedies; 2) miracles, the marvelous interventions of deity; and 3) magic, the use of spells, charms and other impersonal, secret ways. Normally each approach shades into another. The New Testament emerges distinctly different in stressing God's personal presence in healing. This book is scholarly and compressed, yet not ~~to difficult~~ overly technical. For any serious students

1

HEALING IN THE OLD TESTAMENT AND POST-BIBLICAL TRADITIONS

Although the New Testament authors were living, thinking, and writing within the larger context of the Graeco-Roman world, they were all in varying degrees, in overt and subtle ways, influenced by the Jewish tradition out of which Christianity emerged. It is essential, therefore, in assessing the New Testament evidence concerning healing, that we examine as well the biblical and post-biblical evidence concerning health, healing and medicine. The direct and indirect references within the New Testament to this aspect of tradition remind us that these dimensions of the Jewish heritage were indeed present in the consciousness of the early Christians, even though they did not merely reproduce the attitudes and practices of their spiritual ancestors.

1. Stories of healing

Stories of healing are relatively rare in the Old Testament. The first is the curious narrative in Gen 20 of the death threat addressed to Abimelech, who had taken Abraham at his word and acquired Sarah (Abraham's wife) to be his concubine on the basis of Abraham's (half-true) declaration that she was his sister (Gen 20:12). After the deceived king showered Abraham with gifts, the patriarch prayed to God, who healed Abimelech, his wife and female slaves − who had been stricken with barrenness (Gen 20:18). Thus is established a direct cause-and-effect relationship between human disability and divine action. In this case, the inability of the monarch's wives to bear children is the immediate consequence of his having inadvertently violated a divine statute against adultery. As we shall see, this story reappeared in a new form in post-biblical Judaism.

Analogous direct effects of divine judgments on the disobedient or unworthy are evident in the story of Saul's having become disqualified to serve as Israel's king (I Sam 16). Saul's disobedience in failing to destroy the booty captured from the Amalekites results in the Spirit of Yahewh being withdrawn from him and replaced by an evil spirit *from Yahweh* (16:14), which torments him. Saul is advised by his servants to find someone to play the lyre when the evil spirit is upon him, so that "you will be well" (16:16). David is found to perform this role, with the result that "whenever the evil spirit from God was upon Saul", David played the lyre, so that "Saul was refreshed, and was well, and the evil spirit departed from him" (16:23). Both the spirit possession and the remedy for it are provided by God.

The most explicit accounts of healing through a divinely-endowed agent of God appear in the Elijah–Elisha cycles of I and II Kings. There are the story of Elijah's healing of the widow's son (I Kgs 17) and the reports of the death and restoration to life by Elisha of the son of the Shunamite woman (II Kgs 4), and of Elisha's cure of Naaman's leprosy (II Kgs 5). On the negative side of these manifestations of divine power through the prophets are the narratives of the death of Ahaziah, along with the soldiers sent to summon Elijah to help him (II Kgs 1), and the curse of leprosy which befell the greedy Gehazi, who had asked for and received compensation from Naaman (II Kgs 5). There are parallel accounts in II Kgs 20 and Isa 38:16–20 of the sickness of Hezekiah and of his recovery, which is assured by a divine sign (the shadow on the sun-dial reverses direction; II Kgs 20:9–11). His restoration to health is followed, however, by the prophetic announcement of the fall of the dynasty and the captivity of Judah in Babylon (II Kgs 20:16–19). Both the sickness and the healings are manifestations of God's control of history and of human destiny. The achievement of the divine will is effected through the prophet or chosen agent of God.

In Lev 13–14 elaborate procedures are detailed for diagnosing leprosy[1] and for cleansing those who had been afflicted with the disease. It is difficult to determine whether the cleansing process is understood as effecting a cure, or (as is more likely) it constitutes a public declaration that someone is ritually fit for readmission to the Israelite society.[2] The elaborate procedures outlined in Lev 14 include the killing of a bird, the dipping of another bird in its blood, the sprinkling of the blood on the leprous person, and the release of the living bird, apparently as a way of getting rid of the pollution (14:2–9). After the afflicted has shaved off hair, beard, eyebrows, and washed his clothes and his body, he is pronounced clean.

Similar processes are ordered for cleansing the houses of those stricken with leprosy, which confirms the impression that what is being presented here is not the cure of an organic disease but the solution of a problem of ritual impurity that threatens the integrity of the holy people. The method described in Numbers 19, which centres on the burning of a red heifer and the use of the ashes for cleansing purposes, is similar, and confirms the impression that the Levitical Code is not interested in healing the body so much as purifying it, in order to restore it to proper relationship with the people of the covenant. What is involved in Lev 13–14 is not the process of healing leprosy, but the recognition that it has occurred.

2. Signs and wonders

The stereotyped phrase, "signs and wonders", which we have already noted occurs frequently in the New Testament (especially in Acts) with reference to the healing activities of Jesus and the apostles, is widely used throughout the Old Testament and in every type of literature included in that corpus. It is found in various strata of the Pentateuch, from the early chapters of Exodus (Ex 3:20; 4:30; 7:3) through Deuteronomy (Dt 4:34; 7:19; 26:8; 29:3; 34:11). It appears in the earlier (Isa 8:18; Jer 32:20–1; Joel 2:30) and later (Dan 4:2–3; 6:27; 12:6) writings of the prophetic corpus. It is used in the Psalms (78:43; 105: 27; 107:24) and in a late historical writing (Nehemiah 9:10). In most of these occurrences, the "signs and wonders" are identified as God's actions on behalf of Israel at the time of the Exodus and the conquest of Canaan. As Jer 32:20–1 makes clear, however, the term is also used more broadly to recall God's redemptive purpose for his covenant people, and to bear testimony to his control of the events of history which is now evident in the judgment which has fallen on the nation in the form of the Babylonian captivity (32:26–35) and the restoration which God has promised. The phrase also occurs in relation to the signs and portents which confirm Isaiah's prophetic call (Isa 8:18) as well as the signs of judgment that are about to fall, according to Joel 2:30.

The signs and wonders mentioned in Daniel serve two confirmatory purposes: assurance of the vindication of the righteous remnant, as symbolized by Daniel and his companions; and the certainty of God's accomplishment of his purpose in the world (Dan 12:6). The nearest that any of these signs comes to a healing is the pair of occurrences of "signs and wonders" in Daniel, where the faithful are delivered from the fiery furnace and from the lion's den (Dan 3:1–25; 6:27).

In the great majority of cases, even in the Daniel stories, the signs and wonders focus on the destiny of the covenant people, now and in the future. Paradoxically, the prophecies of the healing of individuals in the eschatological future, as described in Isa 35,[3] for example, − the eyes of the blind open, the ears of the deaf are unstopped, the lame leap, the tongue of the dumb sings − are described without the use of the traditional phrase, "signs and wonders". It remained for New Testament writers to link that stylized expression to the healing activities of Jesus and his followers.

3. Yahweh as healer

A central image for depicting God's work in the creation − in what moderns might refer to as both nature and history − is that of healing. Its quasi-metaphorical significance is evident in one of the crucial passages in which the term appears: Ex 15:26. Its position in the book of Exodus is highly significant. Just preceding is the Song of Moses, in which the triumph of God over the enemies of his people and his absolute control of the winds and the waves, as well as of all the tribes of the earth, are affirmed in splendid poetic language (Ex 15:1−18). The themes are echoed in less grand form by Miriam in her prophetic utterance (15:21). The story of the sweetening of the bitter waters of Marah, according to divine inspiration,[4] confirms the picture of God's special care for his people and his utter sovereignty over what we would call the natural order (15:22−5). Following this series of recitals of God's power comes a promise, or more accurately a mutual agreement:

> There the Lord made for them a statute and an ordinance and there he proved them, saying, "If you will diligently hearken to the voice of Yahweh your God, and do what is right in his eyes, and give heed to his commandments, I will put none of the diseases upon you which I put on the Egyptians, for I am Yahweh your healer" (Ex 15:25b−26)

The central purpose of God, this passage implies, is, in accord with his will, to order the human race in general and his own people in particular. That role requires that God act both in judgment and deliverance, in destruction and in sustenance. Thus the earlier chapters of Exodus have recounted how God has sent disasters on those who thwart his purposes or who stand in the way of his plans for his special people. On the other hand, the promise of a reciprocal offer is held out to Israel that if the nation keeps the rules – that is, follows the stipulations for the maintenance of their special identity as the covenant people – God will continue to act in order to enable them to sustain their integrity and their prosperity. That assurance of support for the people ordered by the divine will is portrayed through the image of Yahweh as healer, in contrast to the "diseases" which have fallen on those who oppose him.

Similarly in the Deuteronomic Song of Moses (Deut 32), the opening section, which testifies to God's fidelity and justice (32:4), gives way to an indictment of Israel for its folly and its unfaithfulness to the One who had made a special place for Israel in his purposes (32:6–14), but will call the nation to account for its failure to obey his laws to remain loyal solely to Yahweh (32:15–35). But his plan is not at an end: when Israel has been brought low through God's judgment, then "Yahweh will vindicate his people and have compassion of his servants, when he sees that their power is gone" (32:36), and they are ready to acknowledge the impotence of the false gods to which they had turned (32:37–8). Then they will be ready to acknowledge the unique sovereignty of God, who declares concerning himself:

> I kill and I make alive;
> I wound and I heal;
> And there is none can deliver out of my hand   (32:39)

Once again, it is the figure of healing which is used here to depict God's relationship to his people, in both judgment and vindication.

Similarly, in the earlier prophetic tradition, the relationship of Israel to Yahweh is depicted, both positively and negatively, in terms of healing. Throughout Hosea, for example, the implicit question is raised: who will heal Israel? It is not Assyria that can heal the sickness of Israel and Judah, the prophet declares (Hos 5:13), but Yahweh. When the people return to him, they will be healed by the very one through whom they were "torn" and "stricken" (Hos 6:1). The healing image gives way to that of death and resurrection: "After two days he will revive us; on the third day he will raise us up, that we may live before him" (Hos 6:2). At some points Hosea represents Yahweh in despair over the possibility of Israel's being healed, since her disobedience, her infidelity, her idolatry are seemingly incurable (Hos 7:1–7). Yet so great is the love and compassion of Yahweh for his people, in the past as well as the present, that he cannot abandon them, in spite of their infidelity. Comparing the origins of the nation

with the rearing of a child ("out of Egypt I called my son", Hos 11:1),
the spokesman for Yahweh declares:

> Yet it was I who taught Ephraim to walk,
> I took them up in my arms,
> But they did not know it was I who healed them (Hos 11:3)

Thus the disciplining and the rectification of the people of God are
portrayed under the figure of the divine healing.

The image of God as healer is developed further in Jeremiah. In
Jer 3:22, for example, there is both the plea from Yahweh for the
repentant among his people to return and be healed, as well as the
assurance that the penitent will indeed do so. In 14:19 the prophet
raises the question with Yahweh whether he will indeed heal, since
he has smitten his people: instead of peace has come evil; instead of
healing they have experienced terror. Yet in Jer 30:17–22 is an
elaborate set of promises that God will indeed heal his people, which
divine action is spelled out as including the restoration of their
fortunes, the rebuilding of the city, the increase of their numbers, the
consolidation of the sacred congregation, and a ruler from among
their own number, culminating in the declaration, "And you shall
be my people, and I will be your God" (30:22). This passage leads
directly into Jer 31, which reaches its climax in the announcement
of the New Covenant (Jer 31:31–4), a factor which we shall consider
below.[5]

Two other dimensions of the healing through Yahweh as depicted
by the prophets are (1) the attention paid to the individual person of
piety and (2) the promise of the renewal of nature. Jer 17:5–18 reads
like a psalm, including such features as a divine warning to the one
who does not trust God and the blessing of those that do, and the
glory of the sanctuary as the locus of God's presence in Israel.[6] The
typical psalm-like prayer begins, "Heal me, O Yahweh, and I shall
be healed; save me, and I shall be saved" (17:14). Clearly the healing
imagery is being used in relation to the destiny of the pious individual,
not only to the fate of the nation. The renewal of the human heart
is, of course, an important feature of the New Covenant (Jer 31:33).
The provision announced by Isaiah (19:19–22) for an altar of Yahweh
to be erected in the land of Egypt, which is to serve as a sign and
witness of Yahweh to the Egyptians, will result in the Egyptians
turning to worship the God of Israel and entering into obligations
to Yahweh. The judgment and the redemption of Egypt are described
as Yahweh's "smiting and healing" of the nation, which leads to the

result that "he will heed their supplications and heal them" (19:22). In Ezek 47 the renewal of the people Israel, the central sanctuary in Jerusalem and of the land as a whole will include the transformation of the spring that flows out from the temple mount into a mighty stream, with the resultant change of the dry wady that leads to the Dead Sea into a verdant river valley, and of the Salt Sea itself into a freshwater lake with an abundance of fish.[7] In short, the natural setting of God's people undergoes renewal, just as they do. The image Ezekiel uses in his prophecy of this renewal of nature is "healing" (Ezek 47:8–12).

Two other variations on the theme of God's healing of his people are found in Mal 4:1–3 and Isa 53:4–5. The Malachi prophecy announces the coming of the Day of the Lord, on which the burning of the divine righteousness will consume the "arrogant and evildoers", but the light of the divine presence will be experienced as "the sun of righteousness", which will bring healing, like the rays of the sun. In II Isaiah's servant poem, the servant of Yahweh experienced his rejection and suffering, not as a consequence of his own disobedience, but on behalf of others: "bruised for our iniquities", "wounded for our transgressions", and undergoing "chastisement that made us whole". As a result of this act of God in laying upon him "the iniquity of us all", the prophet tells us that "with his stripes we are healed". Unlike the older use of the image of Yahweh as healer, according to which God sent sickness – that is, judgment – on the disobedient, here Yahweh is transferring to the servant the results of his people's disobedience, and thereby effecting the healing of God's flock (53:6). In distinction from the passages mentioned above, where God acts in unspecified ways to heal his disobedient people, here we are told that it is through a chosen agent, the servant, the bearer of vicarious suffering, that healing is accomplished.

Elsewhere, as in II Chron 7:11–14, the continuance of Israel in the land under the Davidic dynasty is assured, if the nation is both obedient and penitent whenever it fails to obey. There will be pestilences in the land, but humility on the part of the people will bring forgiveness of sin and healing of the land. Similarly, in Psa 103:1–5, Yahweh is the one who forgives the iniquity of his own, and who heals their diseases, with the result that their lives are renewed. In Psa 107:17–22, however, a new dimension is introduced: sickness and affliction are portrayed as the consequences of human sin. Abhorrence of food led some to the edge of death, but when they called upon

God for aid, he delivered them from their plight, "and healed them". Unlike the older levels of the biblical tradition, according to which Yahweh's healing activity is on behalf of the nation and its continuance as God's chosen people, the activity of God in setting things right, or of effecting judgment when things are not right, extends to such personal factors as the sins and the state of health of individuals.

Nevertheless, the motif of healing is found in the later prophetic tradition primarily in relation to the reconstitution of Israel in the New Age. This perspective is already discernible in the oracles of Isaiah of Jerusalem (Isa 30:26), where the renewal and the greatly increased abundance of the land and its resources will take place "in the day when Yahweh binds up the hurt of his people, and heals the wounds inflicted by his bow". In II Isa there is the promise that when God's people begin to care for the hungry, the homeless, the naked, "then shall your light break forth like the dawn, and your healing shall spring up speedily ..." (Isa 58:8). Or again, in a passage both quoted and paraphrased in the gospel tradition (Isa 61:1), the future of Zion is to be transformed through the one anointed by the Spirit, who brings good news to the afflicted and binds up the broken-hearted.

Still more explicit in its use of healing imagery is a passage frequently linked by scholars with II Isa, namely Isa 35, in which the renewal of the land and its people is vividly portrayed, and where the sign of the coming of God to save his people is detailed: "Then the eyes of the blind shall be opened, and the ears of the deaf unstopped; then shall the lame man leap like a hart, and the tongue of the dumb shall sing" (Isa 35:5−6). It will be recalled that there are unmistakable allusions to this passage in Jesus' answer to the questioners from John the Baptist concerning Jesus' mission (Lk 7:22 = Mt 11:4). It is clearly with the aim of demonstrating the continuity between these post-exilic prophetic oracles and the activity of Jesus that Luke describes Jesus as quoting this passage and declaring it to be fulfilled in his work: by the Spirit he has been empowered to preach good news, to proclaim liberation to the captives, and recovery of sight for the blind.[8]

4. Yahweh and the physicians

The only positive account of physicians in the Hebrew canon of scripture is in Gen 50:1−3, where Joseph arranged for the embalming of the body of his father, Jacob, by the Egyptian physicians. Forty days and many physicians were required to complete the task, and then the physicians mourned Jacob for seventy days. Elsewhere in the prophetic, historical, and wisdom traditions, however, physicians are portrayed in strictly negative terms. The useless advice offered by the so-called comforters to Job is dismissed by him as the deceit of liars and the useless prescriptions of physicians. In II Chron 16:11–12, Asa is denounced on the ground that, when he was stricken with a disease of the feet which increased in severity, he did not turn to Yahweh for help but to the physicians. The implication is that Asa got what he deserved by seeking medical rather than divine aid.

On two occasions Jeremiah compares the plight of Israel experiencing exile from the land to a sick child for whom no medical remedy can be provided. The familiar lament of Jer 8:22–9:6 begins, "Is there no balm in Gilead? Is there no physician there? Why then has the daughter of my people not been restored?" (8:22). Using the language that would seem appropriate for a medical examiner, Yahweh declares (Jer 30:12–13): "... Your hurt is incurable, and your wound is grievous. There is none to uphold your cause, no medicine for your wound, no healing for you." This could be read as a metaphorical indication of the grievous condition of the covenant people under the judgment of God, but there is also an implication of the inherent worthlessness of physicians and their effort at cures. That inference is confirmed in the ironic instructions of Jer 46:11, "Go up to Gilead, and take balm, O virgin daughter of Egypt! In vain have you used many medicines; there is no healing for you." A similar note of sarcasm about the physicians is sounded in Jer 51:8, where in the midst of the oracle of doom on Babylon, the advice is offered, "Take balm for her pain; perhaps she may be healed."

The overall import of these passages is that Yahweh is indeed the restorer and orderer of human life, individually and corporately, and no human agency, least of all physicians, can solve problems, alleviate suffering, or cure ills.

5. Yahweh and the magicians

In the patriarchal and the Exodus narratives, magicians and diviners are consulted by the pagan rulers to determine the future and to provide schemes for opposing the divine purposes that are being fulfilled by Yahweh on behalf of Israel. When Pharaoh dreams of the seven fat and seven lean cows and the seven full and seven blighted ears of corn, he consults the magicians and wise men of Egypt (Gen 41:1–8), who are unable to interpret what the ruler has seen. Joseph explains to him that through the dream, "God has revealed to Pharaoh what he is about to do" (Gen 41:25). Similarly in Ex 7–9 there is competition between Yahweh and the wise men, sorcerers, and magicians of Egypt with respect to the plagues which are sent to induce Pharaoh to free the Israelites until a point is reached where the magicians cannot match the powers at work through the God of Israel (Ex 8:18). Using a term which will appear in the gospel tradition in another form, the magicians then tell Pharaoh, "This is the finger of God" (8:19). The powers of the magicians are acknowledged, so that there is no hint of deception or chicanery. What is asserted is the superiority of Yahweh's power to that of the magicians.

In the legal traditions of Israel, various forms of magic are explicitly prohibited. Augury and witchcraft are forbidden, as are practices linked with the dead (Lev 19:26–8). Similar, but more extensive, are the injunctions in Dt 18:10–14 against sacrificing one's children, divination, soothsaying, augury, sorcery, and against mediums, wizards and necromancers. These are "abominable practices before Yahweh", although these types of magicians are widely consulted by the Canaanite peoples. That assessment is attested in Numbers 22–3, where the attempt is made to have Balaam curse the Israelites as they invade the land of Moab, but Yahweh confronts Balaam and dissuades him from saying or doing anything contrary to God's purpose for his people. The only force that shapes the destiny of Israel is God's plan, and no magical practices can thwart that divine intention: "God brings them out of Egypt; they have as it were the horns of a wild ox. For there is no enchantment against Jacob, no divination against Israel; now it shall be said of Jacob and Israel, 'What has God wrought?'" (Num 23:22–3).

In I Sam 6:2 the Philistines try to understand and counteract the baneful effects of the presence of the ark of the covenant in their midst by consulting magicians, who advise sending it back toward Israel, laden with gifts. Among those rulers of Israel who disqualified themselves for the kingly role were Saul, who consulted the witch of Endor (I Sam 28), and Manasseh, who sacrificed his children "practised soothsaying and augury, and dealt with mediums and wizards" (II Kgs 21:6). As a result of these practices, which are attributed not only to the king but to the people as a whole (II Kgs 17:16–18; 21:9–15), the nation is to be taken off into captivity by the Assyrians (II Chron 33:1–13), as a sign of which Manasseh himself was temporarily carried to Babylon as a captive. The practice of magic is pointed to by Isaiah as the ground of the impending judgment (Isa 2–3, esp. 2:6), although God is going to deprive the people of these wicked resources (Isa 3:3). Jeremiah warns against the false prophets and diviners who discount the predictions of divine judgment on the nation (Jer 14:14). He counsels submission to Babylonian domination, contrary to the false advice of "your prophets, your diviners, your dreamers, your soothsayers, your sorcerers" (Jer 27:9) to resist the Babylonians. Similarly, Ezekiel classifies the false prophets of Israel with the diviners who promise peace, rather than the divinely intended judgment. The specifics of the magical practices are provided in Ezek 13:17–18, where there is a pronouncement of "Woe to the women who sew magic bands upon all wrists, and make veils for the heads of persons of every stature in the hunt for souls", followed by a solemn warning against their "delusive visions" and practice of divination (Ezek 13:23). Malachi announces the coming of the messenger who is "to prepare the way before me", whose advent is compared with a refiner's fire and a fuller's soap, and who will move in swift judgment against (among other wicked persons) "the sorcerers" (Mal 3:1–5).

One of the clearest Old Testament instances of magic, and one which is presented by the narrator in a positive light, is the brief narrative in II Kings 13:20–1. There we read that the hasty burial of a dead man on the occasion of an incursion of the Moabites into the land of Israel resulted in the corpse coming in direct contact with the bones of Elisha. The instant result was that the man was brought back to life and "stood on his feet". The automatic effect of the remains of this once-powerful miracle worker seems to shift the incident out of the realm of miracle, where the divine action is invoked or attested. Instead, the story's notion of inherent powers of certain objects is a feature characteristic of magic.

6. The physician as agent of God

A radical shift in attitude toward physicians is evident in Sirach 38:1–15. Instead of being portrayed as an opponent of God, the physician is said to have been created by God and to have provided the medicines "out of the earth" which sensible people will welcome and utilize. His skill leads to justifiable admiration and exaltation; in sharing his knowledge with others he is to be glorified for his wonderful works. In effecting cures the physician is aided by the pharmacist, who prepares the mixtures that cure and relieve pain. As a biblical base for the use of what we might call natural remedies, the writer recalls the story of the bitter waters of Marah (Ex 15:23–5) which were made sweet and potable when Moses threw into the water a tree that Yahweh had shown him. These natural potencies are represented by Sirach as God-given, and were disclosed to the physician in a manner analogous to the advice provided to Moses. Medicines are "created out of the earth" by God (Sir 38:3).

The religious context of healing, according to Sirach, has many features in common with the older perspectives on healing, however. It is ultimately dependent on God, since he is the one who provides the medicines that the physician uses. But prayer and sacrifice are essential for the efficacy of healing. The link between sickness and sin is explicit, so that one should not only purify the heart but also offer generous sacrifices in order to assure the divine favour (Sir 38:9–11). Yet a place must be made for the physician, since he has the crucial role of administering the medicine. Even the physician must pray for divine guidance in the matter of effecting cures and restoration to health (38:14). The curious petition of 38:15 is apparently meant positively rather than ironically:

> As for the one who sins in the sight of his Maker,
> May he fall into the hands of the physician!

Although the sickness is the result of sin, through prayer and sacrifice the ailing one can be prepared for the benefits of the medical aid that the physician has been instructed by God to give. As Geza Vermes has observed, both cause and remedy of the disease are given "through a God-given insight, a kind of revelation, which enables the physician to bring relief to the ailing"[9] (Sir 38:14). Far from their earlier depiction as the opponents of God and his ways, physicians are here presented by Ben Sira as instruments through whom his provisions for human health are available.

How are we to account for this basic shift in attitude toward medicine? The most likely explanation is that Judaism in the Hellenistic period came under the influence of the Greek tradition of medicine which had been developing since before the time of Hippocrates. The impact of Hellenism in this period is obvious in the Jewish adoption of such Greek names as Alexander and Antipater, as well as in more intellectual spheres, such as Jewish adaptation of Stoic ethics and the theory of natural law.[10] It is what might be expected, therefore, that such a basic human concern as healing would likewise be influenced by Greek traditions. The predominant emphasis on herbs and other items readily available in the natural world as the basis of cures recalls the perspective of Pliny in his *Natural History* which we sketched in the Introduction. Although as we observed, Pliny does allow for the healing efficacy of factors which by strict definition would be included under religion or magic, his major emphasis falls on the inherent powers of plants and herbs to enable the body to recover from disorders and resume a healthy existence. What differentiates Pliny's view sharply from that of Sirach, however, is that the former treats the creation as a self-originating, given order, which he simply personifies as Nature, which has been "created – a wonderful subject to contemplate – for the sake of man alone".[11] The access to human welfare lies through the awareness of the first principles of the natural order, which (as we noted above, p. 6) are identified by the Greeks as *sympathia* and *antipathia*. The right use of natural remedies enables human beings to live safely and in health in the midst of the polarities which characterize the natural order.

Sirach, as we have seen, locates the origin of the creation and sovereignty over it with the God of Israel. Healing is achieved by divine revelation, not by natural insight. But in spite of this fundamental distinction, both the positive evaluation of the physician in Sirach and the central importance given by him to remedies available in the created order give evidence of the impact of Hellenistic culture, and specifically of Hellenistic medicine on Jewish thinking in the early second century B.C. Although Pliny was writing in the first century of our era, he looks back to a time centuries earlier when the older Hippocratic tradition, which had a place for natural remedies, was being eclipsed by preoccupation with medical theory and surgical experimentation. Why, Pliny asks, had the use of "simples" been abandoned in favour of medical art which is "lucrative beyond all the rest?"[12] What Sirach describes looks like a Jewish version of a Hellenistic practitioner of natural medicines. As we shall see, the Essenes of Qumran, for all their insistence on withdrawal from society, were even more directly affected by Graeco-Roman medical practice than was Sirach.[13]

7. Sickness and the demonic

Also from the second century B.C. and down into the first century of our era come documents which bear testimony to another view of sickness and healing: the activity of demons and the ability to control them. The Book of Tobit, which was likely written in the first quarter of the second century B.C., links sickness and death with demons.[14]

The author also notes in passing the ineffectiveness of the physicians to meet human needs. Thus, Tobit's blindness, caused by sparrow droppings, could not be cured by the physicians whom he consulted (Tob 2:10), but the cure was effected by the same means − the entrails of a fish − as drove out the demon (6:7; 6:16; 8:1−3; 11:8−14). It is not by chance that the name of the man/angel who guides Tobit to visit his kinfolk, to claim his bride, to drive off the demon that caused her first seven husbands to die on their wedding nights, and that brings him home and enables him to cure his father's blindness, is Raphael: that is, God heals.

In I Enoch 6−11 is told the story of the cohabitation of the fallen angels with beautiful earthly women, and the consequent corruption of the human race through the angels' teaching humankind charms and enchantments (7:1; 8:3) and disclosing the eternal secrets which were to have remained in heaven (9:6). The warning to Noah of the destruction of the race is followed by instructions to Raphael to bind the wicked angels and to prepare them for eternal judgment, even when proclaiming to earth that it will be healed (10:4−7). What differentiates the outlook of I Enoch from that of Tobit on the matter of demonic powers is that Enoch depicts the fallen angels as the adversaries, not merely of human beings, but also of God. They have sought to wrest control of the creation from Him, but their doom in fire, torment and prison is sure (10:13−14).

Jubilees, which probably dates from the middle of the second century B.C., manifests kinship with both Sirach and Enoch. With Sirach, Jubilees shares the notion that medicinal remedies, especially herbs, are part of the created order, and have been revealed to the chosen ones among God's people (Jub 10:10−14). Like Enoch, Jubilees represents the fallen angels, and especially their leader, Mastema, as the instruments that wreak destruction and ruin on disobedient humanity. God, who alone can control these demonic powers (Jub 10:6), removes most of them from earth, but leaves some behind to perform their evil work as instruments of his judgment on humanity (10:7−8). The kinds of acts they perform are detailed in Jub 48, where the plagues that came on the Egyptians were the direct actions of God (48:5−7), while Mastema enabled the Egyptians to carry out their harassment of Moses and the children of Israel. Then the striking statement is made, "The evils indeed we permitted them [i.e., Mastema and the Egyptians] to work, but the remedies we did not allow to be wrought by their hands" (48:10). The dualistic outlook of Jubilees, like that of the New Testament writers, is provisional, however, not absolute. Human ailments and disasters are performed by the demonic powers, but are permitted by God to happen. Ultimately, the powers of evil will be overcome, and the final and eternal restoration of the creation will occur.

Coming down into the first century of our era, we find that Josephus manifests the influence of both Hellenistic medical tradition and of a belief in the link between demons and sickness. In his description of the Essenes in the Jewish Wars (*Antiquities* 8.136) he reports:

> They display an extraordinary interest in the writings of the ancients, singling out in particular those which make for the welfare of the soul and the body; with the help of these, and with a view to the treatment of diseases, they make investigation into medical roots and the properties of stones.

In providing the details of the divine gift of wisdom which Solomon received from God on request (I Kgs 4), Josephus notes that his detailed knowledge of all kinds of creatures, terrestrial and aquatic, of herbs and trees which is evident from his poetry and metaphors attests to his mastery of all forms of nature. All these he studied "philosophically and revealed the most complete knowledge of their several properties" (*Antiquities* 8.44). Thus like the physicians described by Sirach and like Pliny and the tradition which he defends, the welfare of human beings is dependent on knowledge of herbs and other natural items with medicinal potential, to be administered by those, like Solomon, who are knowledgeable in such matters. It is in this tradition that Josephus depicts the medical skills of the Essenes, as well. We shall have occasion below to note some additional evidence from Qumran of direct links between the Essene community there and Hellenistic medical practices.[15]

In his account of the Therapeutae[16] Philo describes the concern of this sect for the health of its members. Not only are all the physically ill cared for within the community, but their cures concern not only the bodies, since they also treat "souls oppressed with grievous and well-nigh incurable diseases, inflicted by pleasures and desires and griefs and fears, by acts of covetousness, folly and injustice and the countless host of other passions and vices". Thus Philo's list of cures undertaken by the Essenes, or Therapeutae of Alexandria, includes what we might call psychic and psycho-somatic ailments as the result of sin, so that more than merely physical medicine is required if true and full health is to be restored.

Josephus' understanding of health is portrayed with other dimensions in his account of the wisdom of Solomon in the passage from *Antiquities* referred to above:

> And God granted him knowledge of the art used against demons for the benefit and healing of human beings. He also composed incantations by which illnesses are relieved, and left behind forms of exorcisms with which those possessed by demons drive them out, never to return.[17]

Josephus goes on to recount an exorcism performed by a Jewish exorcist in the presence of Vespasian. The demon was drawn out through the nose of the possessed man through the use of "one of the roots prescribed by Solomon" (*Antiquities* 8.46–7). Josephus notes that this achievement confirms the reputation of Solomon as one favoured by God and of "surpassing virtue" (*Antiquities* 8.49).

If we invoke the definitions that were offered in the Introduction (p. 3) – medicine as enabling the body to recover its normal state of health through the use of natural medicines and treatment; miracle as healing effected through the intervention of divine power; magic as the achieving of a desired end through the use of efficacious technique or formula – then it is evident that Josephus depicts the Judaism of his time as engaging in all three modes of healing. On the other hand, from the only direct evidence we have of the Essenes (that is, the Dead Sea Scrolls), we can infer the operation there of only medical tradition and miracle, as represented by the performance of exorcisms. In both cases where exorcisms are reported, the factor of forgiveness of sins is operative as well. In the Genesis Apocryphon (IQ GA 20:12–29) there is an account of the healing action of Abraham on behalf of Pharaoh. The cure is effected through the laying on of hands and the resultant expulsion of the plague and the demon that caused it. The control of the demon is described by the use of the term *g'r*, which is the equivalent of the verb widely found in the gospel tradition, and weakly translated as "rebuke", but which conveys the sense of bringing under control a hostile force.[18] The scourges and plagues which came upon the Pharaoh were, as the original Genesis account makes clear (Gen 12:10–12; cf. Gen 20:1–18), the consequence of his having taken another man's wife as his own, even though he did so unwittingly, misled by the woman's husband, Abraham. In this Qumran document, the notion that sickness is the result of sin is complicated by the demon's having come to control the destiny of the Pharaoh. It is in response to the ruler's request for prayer on behalf of himself and his household that Abraham is moved to act, thereby expelling the demon.

A similar diagnosis and cure are described in the Prayer of Nabonidus (4Q Or Nab), where the king has been afflicted with a severe ailment, on the analogy to the loss of sanity by Nebuchadnezzar, according to Daniel 4. The term, *gzry'*, has been regularly translated where it appears in Daniel (Dan 5:7, 11) as "astrologer", but it seems more suitable, in light of the Prayer of Nabonidus to translate it as "exorcist". The euphony of this root, *gzr*, with the technical term for bringing the demons under control, *g'r*, would be more striking if, as seems to be the case, "exorcist" is the actual meaning of the term. What is significant for our purposes is not only the apparent link between healing and demonic exorcism, but also the connection of the expulsion of the demon with the grant of forgiveness of sins. There is in this narrative no hint of magical formula or technique by which the desired result is coerced; rather, the removal of the immediate cause of the ailment (the demon) is accompanied by the granting of forgiveness of sin to the pagan king.

Thus, in spite of differences in detail, the evidence about healing from Josephus, Philo and the Dead Sea Scrolls confirms the picture of a combination of medical practices and belief in miraculous cures among the Essenes. Philo even suggests that the Essenes of Palestine had a kind of welfare clinic for the ailing, when he writes:

> The sick are not neglected [i.e., by the Essenes] because they cannot provide anything, but have the cost of their treatment lying ready in the common stock, so that they can meet expenses out of the greater wealth in full security.
>
> (*Every Good Man is Free*, 87)

Since the factor of cost is prominent in this report about the Essenes, Philo seems to imply that medical aid was sought from outside the community, with the necessity to pay the fees of the physicians. Certainly there is no negative attitude toward medicine, as in the older biblical tradition, even though in the reworking of the scriptural tradition, as we saw in the Prayer of Nabonidus and the Genesis Apocryphon, there is the expectation of divine action through the chosen intermediary of the exorcist. If one brackets the factor of the demonic, the notion of God working through a chosen agent for healing recalls the stories of Elijah and Elisha. But the world-view implicit in the Qumran material includes sharply dualistic features which have no counterpart in the older miracle stories of the biblical sources.

What we see from this survey of the evidence is neither simple continuity of perspective on healing between the Old Testament and Judaism at the beginning of our era, nor across-the-board replacement of the older points of view. The connection between sin and sickness remains. The possibility of divine action, either directly or through an intermediary, to meet the human need is likewise shared by the earlier and the later writings. The differences are the following: (1) medicine comes to be viewed as a positive contribution to human welfare; (2) human suffering and disabilities are regarded as the work of Satan and/or his cohorts. The question arises for the modern historian, how did medical tradition in its approach to human illness achieve such an esteem as to exert broad influence in the Roman world, including not only the more sophisticated of the Jewish population, but even such a culturally withdrawn group as the Dead Sea community? To approach an answer to that question we must look at the development of medicine among the Greeks and Romans in the centuries preceding and following the birth of Jesus.

2

MEDICINE IN THE GREEK AND ROMAN TRADITIONS

The popular esteem in which physicians were held in fifth century B.C. Greece is set forth by Pindar in his *Pythian Ode* (III.47–53) in which he extols the one skilled in medicine who enables:

> those whosoever came suffering from the scores of nature, or with their limbs wounded either by grey bronze or by far-hurled stone, or with bodies wasting away with summer heat or winter's cold [to] be loosed and delivered ... from divers pains, tending some of them with kindly songs, giving to others a soothing potion, or haply swathing their limbs with simples or restoring others by the knife.

Though Pindar is speaking here of Asklepios, it is his role as patron and prototype of physicians that is celebrated. In the *Iliad* (2.728–33) Homer mentions the two sons of Asklepios among those assembled with the ships for the attack on Troy, and in passing notes that they were "good healers both themselves". The implication is that sons carry on the paternal vocational skill: like father, like sons. In the *Pythian Ode* of Pindar quoted above, Asklepios is an extraordinarily endowed human being, who is warned against seeking the life of the immortals. In other traditions, however, Asklepios is both the progenitor of a hereditary clan of physicians, known as the Asklepiads, and the god who comes to the aid of the sick when they visit his shrines, curing their diseases. We shall return to the second aspect of his tradition below when we consider the phenomenon of miracle. Asklepios became, therefore, the god of both the physicians and patients.[1] In some centres of the Greek world, he was honoured as divine healer, while at Pergamum and Cos there were medical schools as well as shrines where the sick awaited his divine visitations.

As far back as the time of Homer, the physician was regarded as a craftsman (δημιουργός, *Odyssey* 17.383) who practised his art in public and for the public benefit. Later, especially in the Roman period, he was to become a functionary within a feudal household. The Greek medical men were free, but often had slaves as assistants. There was no basis for quality control of their services, but presumably the apprentice system that existed helped to regularize procedures and convey knowledge derived from longer experience.[2] In the case of the leading figure in ancient Greek medicine, Hippocrates – or at least in the tradition that attached to his name – there was no cleft between medicine and the ministrations of the gods. As L. Edelstein has observed on the basis of Hippocrates' treatise, *On Regimen* (IV.249–51), everything was believed to have been arranged by the gods. Since nature is divine, so all is divine. There is no need to distinguish human from divine diseases: all are both. The seemingly spontaneous reactions of the body are to be understood as manifestations of divine wisdom.[3] Only later, in Hellenistic times, does a split develop between rational medicine in a religious framework and avowed skepticism, as we shall note below.

At least from the time of Plato on to the time of Galen, physicians in the Greek tradition were widely regarded as philosophers as well as persons possessing medical skills. In the *Phaedrus* (270d ff.) Plato compares the skills of the physician with those of the rhetorician, asserting that the former demands "high and subtle discussion and philosophical speculation about nature", since knowledge of the nature of the soul presupposes knowing universal nature. W. A. Heidel, in his study *Hippocratic Medicine*, observes that in the view of his contemporaries, the name of Hippocrates typified "that rational procedure in the field of medicine which Socrates demands in the theory and practice of oratory."[4] Accordingly, it is assumed that "miracle is to be regarded as a special application of general science, that medicine is the science of the human body as a part of the universe, and that the body is subject to the laws of the universe and is composed of elements (each having its specific character and reactions) common to the body itself and to the world at large".[5]

1. The Hippocratic tradition

Hippocrates did not develop the art of medicine *de novo*, but built on the insights of his predecessors. For example, Alcmaeon (ca 450 B.C.) based his medical theory on the concept of maintaining equilibrium within the body. When a disease or malfunction of the body causes illness, the task of the physician is to identify the cause of the difficulty and compensate for it. He and other pre-Hippocratics concentrated efforts through observation and dissection on one of the bodily functions: Alcmaeon on intelligence and its channels of communication, Empedocles on respiration, Anaxagoras on circulation, Diogenes on flatulence and veins. Herodotus, on the other hand, emphasized the body as a whole. In the Hippocratic tradition from the outset there was a search for general knowledge of the major organs (even though their specific functions were not understood) and of the bones, with less attention given to the veins and nerves. The aim was to discern through practical experience how the various parts of the body functioned, in order to assist the natural curative forces of the body itself.[6]

Medicine in this period relied heavily on the accumulation of information through casebooks, records of plagues, and reports of new species of plants and animals. Diagnosis involved not only the specifics of the individual's symptoms, but also information about race and sex, location, climate, water supply, even social and political conditions. The logic of diagnosis moved from what was discernible to what could be inferred on the basis of generalized knowledge and prior experience.[7] As the Hippocratic tradition continued to develop, medical centres showed preferences for certain analogical bases in diagnosis. For example, the school at Cos based its explanations of disease on biology, while the school at Cnidus made its inferences by analogy with physics. Yet in their theorizing, the physicians in the Hippocratic tradition were handicapped not only by their lack of knowledge of the functions of the major organs – including the heart and the brain – but also by the absence of an appropriate theoretical framework for carrying on their logical analyses. They were limited to such abstract distinctions as hot/cold, wet/dry, vacuum/attraction. The physical basis on which they operated was the grossly inadequate and inaccurate principle of the four elements: fire, air, water, and earth. And they tried to develop features of the human body that would correspond to these in the four humours: blood, phlegm, choler (yellow bile), and melancholy (black bile).

Treatment was aimed at the maintenance of health, primarily through diet and exercise. The medications prescribed were intended to restore the balance of the bodily humours. The evidence scrutinized in making a diagnosis included common nature, the nature of the individual, the disease, the patient's constitution as a whole and in parts, weather, local customs, mode of life, the personality of the patient, and such details as talk, manner, silence, thoughts, sleep or absence thereof, dreams, scratchings, tears, stools, urine, sputum, vomit, earlier diseases, sweat, chills, coughs, sneezes, hiccoughs, breathing, belching, flatulence, haemorrhages, and haemorrhoids.[8]

The art of healing included (in addition to medication, diet and exercise) various factors which in our time would be considered as psychological or psycho-somatic: overcoming worry, candid communication, and the fostering of love for one's fellow human beings and for the arts.[9] As Heidel epitomizes the technique, "Disease was a disruption of natural balance; health was the recovery of it."[10] Heidel expresses a widely-held estimate of Hippocrates in his assertion that this prototypical physician:

> laid the very foundation of science, for the distinction
> between the permanent and the transient, between cause and
> effect, natural or normal and accidental, health and disease
> was clearly apprehended.[11]

That valuation is qualified, however, by the acknowledgment that Hippocrates' reasoning was largely by analogy, and that it was limited by an inadequate grasp of the phenomena as well as by a tendency to oversimplification.[12] Also commonly asserted is the view that Hippocrates sought only natural causes for disease, attributing in merely formulaic fashion sickness or disaster to the gods or to causes beyond human control, with divine intervention depicted only in dreams.[13] When portrayed in this way Hippocrates becomes the model for the post-Enlightenment naturalist, sceptical of all appeals to the divine or to supernatural activity. According to this view, the physician can give an intelligent reason for everything he does (Plato, *Gorgias* 465a) and does everything solely for the good of the whole (Plato, *Laws* 902c). Hippocrates regards the philosophical doctor as the peer of the gods (*De decenti habitu* iv, = ix, 232, Littré).

This rationalistic view of the Hippocratic tradition has been called into question by some recent studies of the history of medicine, however. What has been presented by many earlier historians of medicine as "the facts" about Hippocrates are now regarded as "unverifiable", as "an etiological myth, an analytical scheme dressed up as a narrative of events".[14] Littré's decisions about what to include in the Hippocratic corpus were arbitrary, and have been discredited by more recent discoveries.[15] The chief difficulty, apart from the scattered and fragmentary nature of the Hippocratic tradition itself, is the fact that Hippocrates has been perceived largely through Galen's use of, and comments on, his writing. One may admire Galen for seeking to call his contemporaries back to the classical tradition, as it was found in Plato and Hippocrates, but in doing so Galen was fostering his own reputation as an anatomist and intellect, and in the process was putting down the views of his opponents. The Hippocratic tradition was in Galen's hands not merely a corpus to be expounded but a club with which to beat down his antagonists and detractors.[16] The self-image which Galen sought to project was that of a philosopher–physician who synthesized precise empirical evidence with brilliant theoretical perceptions. As W.D. Smith has shown, Galen in his major medical treatise, *Anatomical Procedures*, "makes an almost ritual gesture toward proving the science is Hippocratic", though what it contains is largely original to Galen himself. He claims to be the sole true heir of Hippocrates, and manoeuvres his enemies into anti-Hippocratic positions. At first Galen evidenced little concern for the question of the authenticity of the Hippocratic material, but later he commented on variants in the text tradition. He suppressed Hippocratic views which were in conflict with his own, polemicized against others who disagreed with him, and concentrated on Hippocrates' surgical works, which were more precise and less controversial. His method was to paraphrase and clarify, with few comments on the opinions of earlier writers, and with a clear aim of dominating the scene with his own "Hippocratic" views.[17] Hippocrates, therefore, and Galen after him (through different versions), scarcely fit the model of scientific objectivity as it came to be venerated in post-Enlightenment western society.[18]

Before turning to an analysis of Galen's attitude toward religion and the impact of his work on the subsequent development of medicine, it is essential to trace the changes in medical tradition in the centuries that separate him from Hippocrates. Hippocrates is given credit for founding the medical school at Cos. Unlike the school at Alexandria, which was largely academic and theoretical in its interests,[19] the 'Ασκληπιάδοι of Cos were a guild, with hereditary membership. Although there is no literary or archaeological evidence, it has been conjectured that in the fifth century at Cos "the training of physicians and the practice of medicine were put on a rational and systematic footing, launching a firm tradition of secular medicine which was never lost in antiquity thereafter".[20] The archaeologist who has given us the fullest report on ancient Cos is at pains to deny there was any connection between the medical school and the shrine of Asklepios that was located in the city.[21] Nevertheless there is a strong likelihood that healing by medical means and by divine intervention went on in centres dedicated to Asklepios, like Cos and Pergamum.[22] The schools at Cos and Cnidos, which seem to have provided the majority of physicians for Greece and later for the Romans, agreed on the centrality of the study of the individual as a means of determining the future course of the disease, but they disagreed as to whether the physicians' main task was to point up the common features (Cos) or to differentiate distinctive features (Cnidos). At Cos the instruction was never institutionalized, as it was at Alexandria, but was in the hands of individual physicians. The dominance of Cos as a supplier of physicians was ended only by the rise of strong competition from schools at Smyrna, Ephesus and especially Pergamum.[23] The successes of these physicians were largely in the realm of external surgical activity, such as dislocations, and cures based solely on observation. The severe limitations under which they worked included not only their ignorance of bacteria as a source of infection, but the absence of human dissection and the dominance of the theory of humours.[24] Standard prescriptions for the ill included diet, baths and exercise.

2. Hellenistic medicine

During the Hellenistic period, physicians were divided in their attitudes toward anatomical research and diagnosis into two groups: (1) the dogmatists, who relied on supposed knowledge of hidden causes (especially of the human constitution and the origins of disease) and who assumed that experience must be supplemented by reasoning and conjecture; (2) the empiricists, who insisted that it was neither legitimate nor necessary to speculate about such matters: "The invisible cannot be known: the doctor's task is to treat individual cases, and for this purpose he must avoid inference and attend to, and be directly guided by, the manifest symptoms of the patient and by these alone."[25] These two different strategies reflect, of course, two different views of epistemology and logic, the one idealistic and the other pragmatic. Although much of the body was only superficially known through the Hippocratic tradition, the information about the sense organs, and especially about the eye, and the blood vessels was remarkably accurate. This developed in part under the influence of Aristotle, and took shape on the basis of analogies between animal and human bodies. Only later did human vivisection become quite common, and only then did more accurate knowledge of the human body begin to emerge. This practice is linked particularly with Herophilus of Chalcedon (270 B.C.) and Erasistratus of Ceos (260 B.C.) who dissected corpses and performed vivisections on condemned criminals.[26] Through vivisection, Herophilus discovered that the brain was indeed the centre of the nervous system, as Plato had conjectured, but he failed to understand the pumping action of the heart. Nevertheless, his major contribution was in the analysis of the pulse: its rate, pattern and pressure.[27]

In a short work of Herophilus' which has survived, the physician gives detailed suggestions for food and drink, month by month throughout the year. In addition to instructions about preparation of the food and baths, he ends each monthly section with advice about how to deport oneself in view of the changing pattern of constellations, including specific days in which certain types of activity are to be engaged in or avoided, including sexual relations.[28] Clearly, then, Herophilus views the human condition not merely in terms of the immediate physical environment and the food and regimen of the body, but considers as essential for human welfare a pattern of life which takes into account the movement of the stars. Curiously, the names for the constellations are not the ones in common usage,[29] but there is no mistaking the fact that astrology is a significant factor in this physician's world-view. Taking into account the gods, as represented by the constellations, is for Herophilus an essential feature of human well-being. His reputation as a leading figure in anatomical science is no doubt warranted, but these rational approaches to medicine seem to have been not in the least incompatible with traditional convictions about the gods and their regulation of human life. It should be recalled that Hippocrates (in *Concerning Airs*, I.8) wrote, "Astronomical knowledge is of great help in the practice of medicine." Galen, on the other hand, was later to ridicule those who attributed influences to the stars, thereby filling their practices with what he considered to be superstitious remedies and puerile precepts. There is no mistaking that in the third century B.C. there were outstanding medical men who stood closer to Hippocrates on this issue than to the more rationalistic position that was to be adopted by Galen. As we shall see, however, even Galen was not wholly consistent on this point.

3. Early Roman medical tradition

In the first century B.C. there was a revival of interest in medicine, and particularly in surgery. Considerable experimentation was carried out with drugs (Heraclides), pharmacology and external surgery (Zopyrus).[30] It is the Roman encyclopaedist, Celsus (fl. in Rome 14–37 A.D.; born *c.* 25 B.C.), however, who is our chief source of information about the development of surgery and anatomy in this period. The impact of Greek medicine was slow in penetrating Roman society. As John Scarborough has observed, the early Romans regarded the gods as supreme lords and governors of all things, so that all events were directed by their influence, wisdom and power. Misfortunes were simply punishment for neglect of the gods. Even the most sophisticated of the Romans, such as Cicero, had a profound feeling for the forces of nature, which were the results of the divine will, and which were mysterious and could only be placated, never understood. These convictions about the *numina* are expressed in Plutarch, *Numa*; and in Cicero, *Laws* and *On the Nature of the Gods*. Even when Greek ideas began to infiltrate the Roman society through the Etruscans, the gods and goddesses of the countryside remained little changed from the earlier native Roman views. The great divinities came to be spoken of in terms of abstractions, but the innumerable divine spirits were thought to have defined activities – some were conceived as personal beings, but most as vague purposive forces.[31]

Yet the influence of Asklepios in Rome may be traced back to as early as the beginning of the third century B.C. It was then, following a plague which struck both Rome and its surrounding countryside in 292, that oracles were consulted, and the advice was rendered that Asklepios should be invited to move from Epidauros to Rome.[32] When the council in Epidauros was reluctant to agree to the transfer, the god appeared and agreed to accompany the delegation to Rome. A serpent from the shrine slid onto the ship, and from the masthead of the ship as it sailed up the Tiber surveyed possible locations for the shrine, choosing finally the island in the Tiber. Significantly, this site is still the location of a hospital, thus preserving continuity with both the religous and the technical aspects of the healing tradition of the Greek god.

Also taken over from the Greeks was the policy of having certain members of the Roman military assigned to administer health services to the army. It is difficult to determine whether there was actually a medical corps, or whether it was simply the policy to assign certain soldiers with knowledge and inclinations to devote themselves to the aid of their fellows. A section of the relief on Trajan's column seems to confirm the second possibility: an ordinary soldier is portrayed there offering medical aid.[33] This was in keeping with the broad Roman practice of learning practical matters from the Greeks, but paying little attention to theoretical questions.[34] Thus Roman technical skill worked to drain the marshes and to provide safe water through the famous aqueducts.

The Encyclopaedists were Roman writers who sought to distil and organize the best of the learning of the past, especially from the Greeks. Chief among these were Varro (116–27 B.C.) and Celsus, whose work on rhetoric, philosophy, law and the military has been lost, but whose compendium on medicine has been preserved, and will be examined in detail below. Varro anticipated the germ theory of disease, based on his observations of the direct link between swamps and disease.[35] Columella (who lived approximately 10–70 A.D.) even went so far as to make a connection between disease and flying insects.[36] Other evidence of the practicality of Romans interested in medicine is tangibly visible in the catheters and forceps which have been recovered from the first century. They are made of steel, iron, bronze, gold, silver and ivory.[37]

4. Celsus

Celsus, who was born about two decades before Jesus and who died three or four years after the crucifixion, was a chronicler of medicine and a collector of information, rather than a creative contributor to medical theory. In the proem to this treatise on medicine[38] Celsus notes that there are three aspects of the medical arts: cure through diet (διατητική), cure through medicaments (φαρμακευτική), and cure by hand (χειρουργία). The empiricists and the theorists he differentiates as follows: the empiricists seek knowledge of the hidden cause of disease; of its evident causes, of natural actions, and of the internal parts. The theorists assume with Empedocles that want or surfeit of one of the elements causes disease, making the following associations with the four elements:

> Fire: hot, rough, red blood, choleric temperament, spring.
> Water: cold, smooth, white phlegm, phlegmatic disposition, winter.
> Air: dry, salt, black bile, melancholic temperament, autumn.
> Earth: moist, acid, yellow bile, sanguine temperament, summer.

The theorists proceed on the basis of reasoned theory, but also draw on information provided through dissection and vivisection, by which means they could watch the bodily processes, and determine the position, colour, shape, size, arrangement, hardness, softness, smoothness, relationships, processes and depressions of each part of the body. Reasoning about treatment is based on this sort of detailed knowledge of the bodily parts, including both theoretical insights and knowledge based on observation.[39]

The empiricists think that general knowledge of nature is unattainable, that the human condition varies according to locale. Not what causes a disease, but what relieves it is most important; diseases are treated by remedies, not by eloquence and abstract learning. The empiricists regard vivisection as cruel and unnecessary, since the exploration of the living person results in death. Celsus himself came down on the side of the theorists, who went beyond analysis of specific ailments to explore the nature of things. The medical investigation must consider not only what caused the disease, but both the bodily condition (humours) and the life-style of the ailing person. He did, however, reject vivisection as cruel.[40] Celsus' work, *De Medicina*, has as its three major themes: (1) How those who are healthy should act; (2) What pertains to disease; (3) What pertains to curing diseases.

The work opens with detailed advice about sleeping, eating, drinking, and bathing in order to gain or retain health; when to force vomiting and purgations; how to treat constipation or loose bowels; how to adjust diet to the seasons of the year (I.3). A curious mix of what we would distinguish as physical and psychological instructions is offered in relation to weaknesses in various parts of the body. For example, the prescription for head weaknesses includes rubbing it, cutting the hair, combing it, frequent walking, avoidance of the hot sun and of hot baths after sweating, using cold water on the head, taking food in moderation, drinking light wine, but also avoiding writing, reading, arguing – even cogitation – especially after dinner (I.4). An indicator of the primarily aristocratic clientele of Celsus is given in his counsel that, when a pestilence comes, one should go abroad or take a sea voyage, or if that is not possible, arrange to be carried about in a litter in order to avoid fatigue (I.10). The effects of the seasons are discussed: summer and the time of the predominantly north wind are the healthiest season; winter and the south wind (off the ocean) are dangerous (II.1.17–21).

Celsus describes in detail the symptoms of a range of ailments, including tuberculosis, dropsy, kidney disease, bladder disorders, and pregnancy problems. The symptoms include pain in the bladder, slimy urine, discharging abscesses, phthisis, dropsy, joint disorders, and epilepsy. Apparently assuming that there is some sort of substance in the body that gives rise to the diseases, Celsus declares: "Every corporeal aid either diminishes substance or adds to it, either cools or warms, either hardens or softens ... Substance is withdrawn by blood-letting, cupping,[41] purging, vomiting, rubbing, rocking, and by bodily exercises of all kinds, by abstinence, by sweating" (II.9). Details of these therapeutic procedures are then presented, including warnings about bleeding – one must take care to cut a vein rather than an artery or sinew – and instructions as to which foods are strong and which are weak (II.16–17), what produces urination, flatulence, and bowel movement and what inhibits them (II.26–33).

The prescriptions for specific diseases begin with the classification, in modification of Greek distinctions among them, as (1) acute; (2) chronic; (3) acute/chronic; (4) curable if treated. Although Celsus rejects the Hippocratic theory that diseases must be treated in accord with the designation of the most critical days of the sickness period (third, fifth, seventh, eleventh, fourteenth, twenty-first) on the ground that Hippocrates and his contemporaries were taken in by Pythagorean theory about numbers, he does suggest a pattern of treatment: only water is to be given for the first two days, followed by alternate days when water is given one day and wine the next; the patient is to be kept awake during the day, and given only minimal liquid and such food as is absolutely necessary to sustain strength (III.4). He sketches detailed correlations between the pattern of fever and the giving of food, on the assumption that the body rejects food when it is not needed, but demands drink when to take liquid is most dangerous (III.5). For nearly all internal diseases – including those that in our time would be differentiated as infectious or organic – the prescribed treatments consist of baths, enemas, emetics, bloodletting, diet, liquids, and sweating or cooling. What might be called even today "home remedies" are also part of Celsus' repertoire, from mustard to chicken broth (III.16; IV.17).

The anticipations of psychotherapy which we noted above become even clearer when Celsus is prescribing for treatment of insanity and kindred mental disorders. Standard therapy included shaving the head, exciting the patient to sneezing, pouring rose oil on the head and in the nostrils, applying herbs and rubbing the body. If the victim is manic or depressive, his or her disposition is to be offset by stern rebuke or by playing music in the patient's hearing. There is a qualification, however: "More often ... the patient is to be agreed with rather than opposed, and his mind slowly and imperceptibly is to be turned from the irrational talk to something better." Interest is to be aroused in other matters, through reading aloud, through having the patient recite something retained in the memory, or by inducing eating by placing the ailing one on a couch in between those who are dining. In addition to drugs and fetishes to induce sleep, rubbing, rocking and exposure to the sound of falling water are recommended. A more radical proposal is trepanation. In case of melancholia, weak food is to be ministered, and there is to be a removal of all causes of fright, counteracted by the raising of hopes. Entertainment is to be offered through story-telling and games. Any work that the patient has done is to be set before him or her and publicly praised. At the same time, the depression should be reproved and depicted as being without a cause, the point being made that in the very things which are being interpreted by the patient as trouble there is in fact a cause for rejoicing rather than for solicitude (III.18).

If the patient's mind (*consilium*) is out of touch with reality, then treatment by torture is to be administered: starvation, flogging, fetters, sudden frightening, fatiguing exercise, and denial of fat or wine in the diet. Victims should not be left among those they do not know, or among those whom they despise or disregard. A change of scene is recommended, and even when the mind returns, there should be journeys at least once a year (III.19). A similar mix of physical and psychic elements of treatment is apparent in the prescription of what is to be avoided by epileptics: sunshine, bath, fire, cold wine, sexual relations, overlooking a precipice or anything terrifying, vomiting, fatigue, anxiety, and all business. The last resource for the insane and the epileptic is to let blood from both legs near the ankle, incise the back of the scalp and apply cups, burn the back of the head just below the highest vertebra "in order that the pernicious humour may exude from the burns" (III.23). Clearly for Celsus the fundamental factor in the treatment of disease is provided by his doctrine of the humours, however close he may have come in some ways to the modern perspectives of psycho-somatic medicine.

At a number of points in his compendium of treatments for human disease, however, Celsus borders on the realm of magic. His counsel for treating those with fantasies is a case in point: those who are depressed are to be given black hellebore as a purge; those who are manic are to be administered white hellebore as an emetic (III.19–20). W. G. Spencer has correctly recognized in this and similar practices of Celsus the impact of imitative magic. Other examples are the consumption of ox spleen to aid an enlarged spleen and of boiled worms to rid one of ear maggots.[42] In the midst of a string of prescriptions for diseases of the throat and abdomen in Book IV Celsus notes, in passing, "I hear it commonly said that if a man eat a nestling swallow, for a whole year he is not in danger from angina" (IV.7). Or again, after describing a concoction made from turpentine resin for the relief of constricted breathing, Celsus observes that it is "not a foolish idea that the liver of a fox should be dried, pounded and the mash sprinkled on the above [mixture], or that the lung of the animal, as fresh as possible, roasted without touching iron in the cooking, should be eaten" (IV.8). Similarly, when one has been bitten by a scorpion, one should pound it up and eat it (V.31).

The dimension of medicine in which Celsus more nearly approximates modern medicinal insights and understandings involves treatment of wounds, broken bones, and ailments of the lower abdomen. In Book VI he describes and prescribes for the treatment of wounds, most of them inflicted by weapons. He notes those conditions under which recovery from a wound is impossible: when either the base of the brain, the heart, the gullet, parts of the liver, or the spinal marrow has been pierced; when the middle of the lung or the small intestine or stomach or kidneys have been wounded; or when the arteries around the throat have been cut (VI.1). He advises against tampering with internal wounds, "unless it be to cut away some bit of liver or spleen or lungs that hangs outside. Otherwise internal wounds will be healed by the regulation of diet, and by those predicaments which I have stated in the preceding book to suit each individual organ" (VI.26).

In the case of dropsy, the physician is to let the liquid out by cutting into the abdomen, avoiding the blood vessels, and inserting a tube for drainage, until it is no longer needed and can be removed. Extrusion of the intestines is to be handled by thrusting them back through the wound, unless it needs to be enlarged. His advice about rupture of the abdominal walls, especially around the genitals, discloses an astonishingly accurate knowledge of the anatomy of these organs. His instructions include operations on the penis, adjustments of the foreskin, and aid for the inability to urinate. Likewise remarkable is the procedure for the removal of kidney stones, which involve elaborate precautions for restraining the patient (there being no anaesthetic, of course), manipulation of the stone(s) by the hand of the surgeon inserted through the anus so that the stone comes to the mouth of the bladder, whence it can be removed by a special surgical device. If there is consequent bleeding, the patient is to be given a seated bath in strong vinegar. If urination does not occur the next day, the surgeon is to reinsert his hand and stroke the bladder so that the hindering blood clot may pass through.

Similar procedures are suggested for problems of the vagina and uterus, including the closure of the entrance, the death of the foetus, the determination of its position, and the difficulty when the womb opening contracts. There are descriptions of a hook that should be used to remove a dead foetus, and instructions about dissecting the foetus if necessary. With regard to broken bones and bone diseases, Celsus offers detailed advice. After giving the symptoms of bone disease, including ulcers and fistulae, he explains how the surgeon is to expose the diseased area, cauterize it, and scrape it until the white bone is reached. Other details of treating bone ailments include removing, cutting, boring, and excising the bones; this is followed by advice as to how the healing may be promoted, and how to reunite broken bones, such as setting a collar bone or treating broken ribs. The procedures are the basic and obvious ones: stretch the bones into the correct position, apply splints and bandages, and slings where appropriate. When gangrene sets in, only amputation is possible. One should refracture limbs which have been shortened by improper treatment. His proposals for dislocations seem compatible with modern methods, and include such obvious warnings as the dire consequences of spinal injuries.

Considerable space is devoted in Bk VI.5 – 6 to analysis and treatment of diseases of the eye and ear – both of which figure prominently in other healing accounts from the first century: e.g., the gospel narratives. Eye infections are to be treated by keeping the ailing one in a dark room, withholding food, and by administering blood-letting and a clyster. Various salves were prescribed for growths and severe eye infections, including trachoma, ophthalmia, cataracts and functional disorders. For decline in eyesight, the sufferer is told to walk and exercise a great deal, to bathe frequently with rubbing over the whole body, and with application of iris unguent to the head. After this, when the subject is sweating, he or she is to be wrapped up and to remain covered until reaching home. In the following days acrid foods and a gargle of mustard are prescribed. Injuries to the eyes from outside are to be treated by anointing the eyeball with the blood of a pigeon, swallow or dove. Diseases of the ear are to be treated early, since to neglect them may lead to madness and death. Prescriptions include spices, vinegar and wine, as well as poultices and liquids dropped into the ear (VI.7). A similar list of remedies — including rubbing, baths, diet, enemas, poultices, gargles, blood-letting, and plasters — is offered for such disorders as ulcers in the mouth or throat, a prominent navel, diseases of the genitals and the anus.

Celsus neatly epitomizes his attitude toward medicine in the proem to Bk VII of his *De Medicina*:

> The effects of [surgical] treatment are more obvious than any other kind; inasmuch as in disease luck (*fortuna*) helps much, and the same things are often salutary, often of no use at all, it may be doubted whether recovery has been due to medicine, or a sound body or good luck ... But in that part of medicine which cures by hand, it is obvious that all improvement comes chiefly from this, even if it be assisted somewhat in other ways.

Celsus is expressing himself here in terms which might be regarded as those of a pragmatist with a strong admixture of Roman traditionalism. He has nothing to say about the gods, either those of the Roman pantheon or the immanental power and purpose of *pneuma*, as one finds it in the Hellenistic thinkers, particularly those of Stoic persuasion. The Roman belief in the somewhat vague but omnipresent *numina* seems to be implied by his confidence in folk remedies and by evidences of homeopathic and sympathetic magic which are discernible throughout his treatise on medicine. What is missing is the presence and power of a healing divinity like Asklepios. Instead one finds a pervasively pragmatic attitude toward healing, with traces of folk beliefs sprinkled throughout. Thus our best-preserved source for knowledge of Roman medicine in the early first century of our era fits well with the picture one gains from the historical sources of the political rulers: deferential to the tradition, at least for public relations purposes, but dedicated chiefly to what produces results.

5. Dioscorides

Celsus' public career seems to have ended with the death of Tiberius and the accession to power of Caligula; the *floruit* of Dioscorides apparently began with Claudius' coming to power and seems to have ended with the death of Nero. The medical encyclopaedia of Dioscorides is known as the *Greek Herbal*,[43] though that is scarcely an adequate indication of the contents of the work. Its five books describe the medicinal values not only of herbs, but also of oils, ointments, trees, animals, fish, reptiles, insects, human effluences and excreta, cereals, roots, juices, saps, vines, wines – even fresh and salt water! – metallic ores and stones, condiments and such cooking items as olive oil and vinegar.

The description of the medical value of these substances includes details of the appearance of each, its place of origin, instructions about the proper harvesting and preparation of each for medicinal purposes, as well as warnings about the dire results of false identifications and overdoses. For the most part, the ailments to be treated by these various means are internal to the body, concerned with organic malfunction. But intrusive factors are also considered frequently, such as the bites of serpents, scorpions and other venomous creatures. In some cases, however, the medication is not taken into the body or even applied to it directly, as in the case of an ointment, but is hung around the neck, or used as an amulet, or placed in a window, or the body is to be struck with it. One benefit of some of these medications, as we shall examine in some detail below, goes beyond what in modern times would be considered the realm of medicine to include the warding off of witches, demons and enchantments.

Although Dioscorides' opening justification for having compiled his *Greek Herbal* may sound vague, it is actually significant in that it reveals his basic outlook on medicine and, in some sense, on human existence. He declares in the opening section of his work that this treatise is necessary because it is linked with and contributes greatly to "the whole art of healing". The explicit contribution of the medicines is, of course, the substance of what follows in his compendium, but what is implied is that human existence is only in part under the influence of the internal organic processes and the introduction into the body of the substances which can ease or improve or aid the healthy functioning of those processes. What he assumes those other forces to be which shape and directly affect human life is only hinted at or disclosed in passing. There is no direct place given to the gods in the traditional sense, although superhuman forces appear at significant points throughout his treatise. At times his remedies border on the magical, at other times on the religious. They are not limited, therefore, to what one might call, in the spirit of the Enlightenment, purely scientific data.

Typical of the linked descriptions/prescriptions, of which there are more than 600 in the *Greek Herbal*, is the first, concerning *Iris illyrica* (I.1). After describing the physical appearance of this type of iris, he notes that it has a warming effect on the body, which makes it suitable for the treatment of coughs and of humours that are "hard to bring up", as well as for purging thick humours and choler. Drunk with vinegar, iris serves as an anti-toxin against "venomous beasts". It aids women having menstrual difficulties and persons stricken with sciatica, ulcers, headache or sunburn. In an understandable understatement he adds, "In general they [i.e., iris plants] are of very much use." Other ailments and the medication effective for them are *Meum* for urine blockage in children (I.3), *Kardamon* for kidney stones (I.5), and *Nardus* for nausea and flatulence (I.6). Cinnamon overcomes darkening of the pupil of the eye (I.13); *Amomum* eases pain and aids sleep (I.14); *Kostos* relieves difficulties of the uterus and helps in case of snakebite (I.15). *Kankamon* has a wider range of benefits: it helps one to lose weight and is good for epilepsy and asthma, for rotting gums and toothache (I.23). Olive oil is presented, not as an ingredient for cooking, but as an emetic and purge in case of poisoning or constipation, as well as an aid in getting rid of worms (I.30). Wild olive oil, however, will keep away grey hairs, if applied daily (I.31). Another cosmetic aid is oil of radish, which helps cure pimples (I.43). Unguents include oil of laurel (I.49), which will ease discomfort in joints and sinews, or oil of cuperas, which relieves stiff necks (I.65), while the juice of the acacia thorn will dye hair black and tighten up loose joints (I.133). Oil of myrtle acts as an anti-perspirant (I.48), as does *Oleum homotribes* (I.29).

Some of the features of this material strike one as simply representing perennial values, while others display some resemblances to healing stories in the gospel tradition. Two of the gifts of the Magi are included: frankincense and myrrh (I.81; I.77), which are both described by Dioscorides as medicaments. The former is said to stop bleeding, cure malignant ulcers, ear problems, spitting blood and difficulties with female breasts. If drunk by those who are healthy, however, frankincense causes madness. Myrrh, if of the proper sort, grown in Arabia, and if properly prepared, helps with problems of the vulva and menstruation, and with protracted coughs, the ague, bad breath, broken bones, impetigo, falling hair, ulcers of the eye, and darkened pupils.

On the other hand, Dioscorides describes as beneficial certain items which are mentioned in the New Testament, but which would have been repulsive to Jews as well as to most early Christians. For example, the dust, debris, clippings and parings left behind from the human bodies in gymnasia and baths, when applied as salve, aid stiff joints, abrasions and old ulcers. Clearly these are examples of sympathy/antipathy of the kind mentioned by Celsus.

In Book II of the *Greek Herbal*, where the medical value of living creatures is under examination, the powers of blood, both human and animal, are presented (II.97). Blood from certain birds heals the eyes; blood of goats, deer and rabbits stops dysentery and fluxes. Not surprisingly, dog's blood cures hydrophobia – another instance of cure by sympathetic means. The blood of the tortoise relieves epilepsy. Menstrual blood, however, renders those who touch it infertile (antipathy?), but anointing with it eases gout and erysipelas (II.97). Similarly, the drinking of a potion of wine mixed with goat dung cures jaundice, while at the same time it causes abortions. A mixture of wine and dry pig dung relieves throwing up blood and pains in the side. For children, mouse dung administered as a suppository has an emetic effect, while dog dung, if collected during dog days, stops the bowels (II.99). Drinking one's own urine is a remedy against the bite of a viper, while boar urine removes stones from the bladder, and bull urine eases an ear ache.

There is no hint in any of these medical descriptions of the problems of purity that are important in the biblical tradition (Leviticus 11–15) and which are presented as an issue between Jesus and his opponents in the gospel tradition. What is at stake in the gospel narratives is not merely the effectiveness of the healing, but also the standing of the person who is ailing and then healed within the covenant community. Values are attached to certain items in the gospel tradition in ways utterly different from those of the medical tradition that Dioscorides is reporting. For example, honey is the food of John the Baptist as the ascetic diet of the true prophet (Mk 1:6; Mt 3:4), while in Dioscorides' account, honey in certain mixtures is of value in such a range of ways as killing lice and nits, easing surgical problems in circumcision, healing sore tonsils and quinsy (II.101). The presuppositions which lie behind these two bodies of tradition are significantly and basically different, even though both are concerned for human welfare.

John Goodyer included in his seventeenth-century English translation of Dioscorides' *Greek Herbal* references to witches and demons, against which certain plants are said to provide protection (e.g., III.156; IV.58). These passages are not found in the manuscripts used by Max Wellman in preparing his critical edition of Dioscorides, and are very likely Byzantine additions. Yet even in the older and presumably more reliable manuscript tradition there are frequent claims of the efficacy of certain herbs and other materials as amulets, as protection against certain types of disabilities, and as love philtres. For example, *Scilla*, if hung in front of the door, wards off poisons (II.202). *Lepidum latifolium* relieves toothache if hung about the neck (II.205), while *Dipsacus sylvestris* when hung about the arm or neck protects against quartan fever (III.13). *Aporine*, if hung in a purple cloth, drives off the ailments that beset cattle (III.105). *Asplenon*, if hung about the neck, acts as a contraceptive, and is especially effective if combined with the spleen of a mule. The acme of efficacy is achieved, however, if the plant has been dug up on a moonless night (III.134). The absence of the moon and the potency of a part of the body of the barren mules show that the influence of sympathetic magic is a significant factor in what otherwise reads as a series of straightforward medical proposals.

What would today be called psychological effects are also described by Dioscorides. Hanging *Leontopodion* (IV.128) and *Katanke* (IV.131) around the neck causes them to act as love philtres, while jasper stone functions in general as an amulet, but when worn around the thigh, facilitates in the delivery of a child. *Melitites* is a multi-purpose amulet: when carried by a servant, it improves relationships with his master, causing the latter to forget failures or misdeeds on the servant's part. It facilitates production of milk by goats and sheep as well as by human mothers. When placed around the neck of infants, it improves their health, their dispositions and their chances of surviving. Further, it predisposes kings and judges to be favourable toward those who carry it, since it imparts a gracious air to its bearers (V.133).

There are also explicitly religious dimenisions of the uses of some of these herbs, plants and other substances, according to Dioscorides. It is important, as he represents it, to maintain good relationships with the divinities and to match one's actions to the astrological conditions as well. At the end of long instructions about the medicinal uses of *Litharge* (*Spuma argendi*) and about how to prepare it for medical use, he notes, "After placing it on a new earthen platter and draining off all moisture, set it in the sun for forty days under the Dog Star, and having dried it, use it" (V.87). Hellebore, which figures so importantly in the medication prescribed by Celsus, is said by Dioscorides to have a multitude of beneficial effects: on epilepsy, melancholy, arthritis, paralysis; it eases menstrual problems and aborts a foetus; it improves hearing, cures psoriasis, impetigo and forms of leprosy; and it relieves a toothache. Planted near vines, it causes them to produce grapes which, when made into wine, act as a purgative. But its effects are also said to include the warding off of evil from houses. Dioscorides advises that while the plant is being dug up, the digger is to pray to Asklepios and Apollo, while observing the flight of the eagles. Great precaution must be taken, however, to avoid allowing the birds to see one harvesting the plant, since if they see the diggers at work, the death of the workers will result. The work must be done in haste, while the diggers eat garlic and drink wine as a safeguard against the powerful effects of the hellebore (V.162).

Clearly, the efficacy of this and other herbs is not purely physical, nor are the forces at work through these herbs and substances merely digestive or biological. Rather Dioscorides' understanding of the cosmos includes careful attention to such predictive and portentous factors as augury based on the flight of birds. These dimensions which transcend the realm of nature, together with elements of magic and astrology, as well as aspects of both traditional veneration of the classical gods and folk religion, are blandly woven together in this handbook of medical art in the first century. When one notes that Dioscorides was part of the imperial establishment in the later decades of the Julio-Claudian dynasty it is clear that in the centre of power, healing was not regarded as merely a product of what might today be called pure science.

6. Medical practice among the Essenes at Qumran

As we observed earlier (pp. 23–25) mention of ailments in the well-known Qumran documents is limited to occasional references to exorcisms, as in the Genesis Apocryphon and the Prayer of Nabonidus. These passages will be further analysed in the discussion of miracle in Chapter 3. But the astonishing fragment from Qumran Cave 4, mentioned above, which has recently been published, gives clear evidence of knowledge there of Hellenistic medicine, and perhaps even of the presence within the community of a kind of health officer who treated both members of the community and visitors. In what appears to be a medical report to his superior (perhaps the prior of the community), one Omriel describes the ailments of persons at Qumran – possibly outsiders who were there only temporarily – and how he sought to heal them.

The brief document, which has been given the designation 4Q

Therapeia, includes terms taken over directly by transliteration from the Greek. This indicates both knowledge of and conformity to contemporary first-century medical practice of the Hellenistic– Roman variety in terminology, diagnosis, and prescription. This document is for the first time made available in a scholarly edition in the appendix of this volume, which was prepared by James H. Charlesworth on the basis of photographs of the fragments published by J. M. Allegro in his sensational *The Dead Sea Scrolls and the Christian Myth* (New York: Prometheus Books, 1984; repr. of 1979 U.K. ed). Since the manuscript is sadly deteriorated, it can be read only through infra-red photographs, with the result that further careful study is essential in order to reach assured readings. But the basic nature of the document as evidence of the medical activity in the Dead Sea community is agreed upon by Allegro and Charlesworth, even though they differ in details of their reconstructions, and thus in the meaning of the text.

There can be no doubt as to there having been wide knowledge of medicine in the Hellenistic tradition among Jews of first-century Palestine, since that perspective on sickness and health can now be shown to have penetrated even such a remote counter-cultural community as Qumran. And if Charlesworth's proposal that the document was one of a large series of periodic reports to the monastic superior is correct, then we can be sure that the medical view of disease and disorders was shared by a group that also looked directly to God for solution of its problems – that is, its members both practised medicine and believed in miracle. The suggestion that this document is a medical report calls to mind one of the treatises written by the next person whose work we shall examine: Rufus of Ephesus, from whom has been preserved a journal in which he reports his care of the sick.

7. Rufus of Ephesus

A major source of knowledge of Roman medicine in the middle of the second century is Rufus of Ephesus (ca 110–180). In addition to the standard edition of his surviving works,[44] there has recently come to light an Arabic translation of his *Journal of the Sick*, in which he describes in detail how he diagnosed and prescribed for patients who were brought to him for treatment.[45] Especially from this recently-discovered work it is possible to see how he continued in the tradition represented by Celsus and Dioscorides, but with certain modifications along theoretical lines. In Sec. III.8 of the *Journal* he observes that the correction of an imbalance of the temperaments (κράσις) is "the most important therapeutic means, since it is δυσκρασία which produces such a humour, and the production of the humour comes to an end only through the correction of the temperament."[46] The implicit link between organic and what we would call psychological aspects of the human being has now been made explicit. The temperaments are identified with blood, phlegm, yellow and black bile, and these in turn produce the humours which are now referred to as "sickness material". For the most part, recovery can occur only when the sickness material has been removed, but occasionally Rufus sees healing as taking place simply when the temperaments have been balanced (VII.20–1). Throughout the *Journal* he describes the removal of the sickness material by means of blood-letting, defecation, and specific medication – in decreasing order of frequency of prescription. At the same time, he deals more explicitly than his predecessors with the psychological aspects of the temperaments, especially of melancholy: fear of death, for which play and pastimes are prescribed (II.16); mild fear of death, combined with the struggle to master geometry and involvement in the economic affairs of the aristocracy (III.1); the anxieties of a man rescued from drowning (IV.1); guilt of a man over having severely injured his sexual organs and thereby his possibility of sexual gratification (V.1). Treatment involves removal of the sickness material: "It accords with the laws of nature, that once a part of the burden of the weight of the congestion has been removed, the rest will come out as well" (VI.17). On the other hand, a young man with a head ailment of a type from which recovery is rare was treated by an application of fragrant juices to his head, and thereupon began to recover. Rufus remarked, "It was a miracle that he recovered without a letting, but that was because his ailment was the result of imbalance of the temperaments (δυσκρασία), not the presence of a sickness material" (VII.1–21).

Another of Rufus' preserved essays is *Concerning the Interrogation of the Sick*.[47] Questions must be asked of the patient in order for the physician to know what is associated with the disease and to be able better to treat it. First, the sick person must be interrogated in order to determine if the sickness is real rather than imaginary, what the patient's strengths and weaknesses are, and in what members of the body the disorder is lodged. Note is to be taken of the clarity, cogency and consistency with which responses are offered by the patient.

For example, was the patient deaf before the disease came? Or is it a consequence of the illness?

Important for Rufus' diagnostic process is whether the illness shows evidence of melancholy: without melancholy, the symptoms are hoarseness, crippling of the tongue, ailments of the chest and lungs; with melancholy, one expects great energy and overwhelming depression. If the ailing one is forgetful or inarticulate, one may expect either a high fever or epilepsy, or even delirium. Chest diseases will be readily recognized when there is roughness of voice, pleurisy, catarrh, or loss of breath. The search for diagnostic clues should include inquiry of those accompanying the patient, especially in the case of a child, an elderly person, or one who speaks another language. Interrogation of the patient is of little value if the disorder is lethargy, catalepsy, speechlessness, deafness, or extreme weakness. The direct cause of the difficulty may be determined in the case of dog or reptile bites, or wounds, but sometimes the patient will not be aware of the cause of the ailment, as in the case of a blow to the head.

Inquiry should also be made as to whether the symptoms are recent or chronic, and if recurrent, what has helped in the past. Information is needed about medications taken, about eating habits, about favourite dishes. Thus Rufus seeks to combine insights from wide past experience with the specifics of the situation of the patient. If the illness can be shown to be the consequence of external forces, it is far easier to treat than if it is the result of inner, invisible factors. In a section dealing with dreams, Rufus testifies to their diagnostic significance, as in the case of a boxer whose trainer told him to ignore a warning that came in a dream, with the result that the boxer developed chest pains and shortness of breath − what would be seen today as typical symptoms of cardiac difficulties − and died.

In the course of outlining his diagnostic method, Rufus defines his position in relation to the Hippocratic tradition. Although he rejects the charge of his critics that he is anti-Hippocratic, he objects to the claim of Hippocrates that, on arrival at an otherwise unknown city, he could determine the water supply, the seasons, the typical diet, the epidemic diseases, and the patterns of childbirth. Rufus acknowledges how much he has learned from Hippocrates (from this "the best of all doctors") but he wants to supplement and refine that knowledge by his own strategy of inquiry: "I advise anyone who wants to arrive at correct knowledge of everything, not to take a position over against inquiry."[48] Local peculiarities and customs must be taken fully into account in diagnosis, since human nature is not the same everywhere.

From the series of test cases which Rufus recounts in his *Journal*, we may examine in detail two in which the ailment is similar to that of persons who are described in the gospels as coming to Jesus for help, and a third which has no counterpart in the Gospels: a case in which the death of the patient is a foregone conclusion in the mind of Rufus. Two of these case-studies in which the ailment is similar to those of persons brought to or encountered by Jesus concern epileptics. The symptoms of the boy brought to Jesus in Mk 9:14–29 – a dumb spirit, which seizes and dashes him to the ground, and the foaming at the mouth, and the grinding of his teeth – are perhaps universally recognized as indicators of epilepsy. The case is less clear in Mk 1:23–6, in which a man is under the control of an unclean spirit which convulses him. The case histories of Rufus' *Journal*, to which the editors have assigned the numbers XV and XVI, describe both epilepsy and its cure. One man has epilepsy, localized in his hand. When the hand was bound to his side, a cure resulted. Another had the disease centred in his knee, and recovered with the application of oil and massaging. A third was treated by having his head rubbed with oil as an attack was impending, with the result that the attack was delayed for three hours, and after regular treatment, recovery was complete.

The fullest account of a cure of epilepsy describes a case which was located in the stomach. The victim, who was forty years old, was required to sit through long meetings, which delayed his meals, and which brought on a sense of dizziness. Rufus opined that rough humour was collecting in his stomach, which then became acid and burning. The prescription of bitter gourds by another doctor, who thought a phlegmatic condition was to blame for the disease, brought on the shakes and restlessness. Rufus detected the characteristics of melancholia and ordered him to take white barleycorn cold, in order to counteract the black bile. In addition the patient was to eat goat and cow thighs, cooked with barleycorn. The delay in his meals was seen by Rufus as the cause of his constipation, for which Rufus prescribed a suppository, as well as a lighter, moist diet, which would thin out the sickness material. Through this treatment and other purges over a period of fifty days, a complete recovery was achieved. A permanent rule, however, was to avoid delaying meals and to include warm water and bread.

Case XVII in Rufus' *Journal* depicts a woman stricken with paralysis, which was complicated by bleeding from the uterus. The details correspond to features of the story of the paralytic in Mk 2:3–12 and that of the woman with the haemorrhage in Mk 5:25–34. Even the detail that efforts by physicians other than Rufus to resolve her difficulties of breathing and bleeding made her worse rather than better match the plight of the woman with the bloody issue (Mk 5:26). Rufus diagnosed her condition as "a hot, dry δυσκρασία", resulting from her having eaten too much dry, warming food. He prescribed a salve of deer fat, styrax, oil and wax to be applied to her neck, but difficulty with breathing continued. When this woman, whom he describes as "scrawny", became his exclusive responsibility, he shifted the treatment to a wax salve made with rose oil, honey and bees wax. Evenings she was required to eat fish, turnips, butter and curds cooked in a soup. The wax salve was changed each night, and the diet continued, with the addition of mixed wine, and evening baths. The result was gradual improvement and ultimately, complete recovery.

Evident in the writings of Rufus is the shift toward increasing complexity in the treatment procedures, including the use employed by the physicians of surgical equipment. For instance, in his essay *On Kidney and Bladder Ailments* Rufus describes the instruments and surgical procedures for removal of stones from the bladder.[49] Rufus adduces in his *Journal* a detailed exhibit of the soundness of his rule that no one regains health when there is an inflammation of the inner throat, unless the infection is in the gums and is small. A young man brought to Rufus had inflamed gums and shortness of breath with severe pain. The throat itself was not inflamed, however. After warning the patient's companions that chance of recovery was not good, he withdrew two units of blood, which seemed to free his breathing. But Rufus was reluctant to draw any more, for fear that the man might faint. After five days he administered an enema, and then began strengthening the man with powerful perfumes. He did not use a compress or gargle, since even such powerful methods cannot suppress an inflammation of this type. Indeed Rufus feared that it might be impossible to force such potent sickness material from the man's body. More bloodletting eased the breathing further, but did not alleviate the pain. Day by day the breathing eased, and the bloodletting continued. With this development, Rufus's hopes rose, and he ordered the patient to gargle with berry juice and spices. The breathing became still easier, and he prescribed a bath in water containing seeds and juice, barley and coriander. Soon the man could swallow, and was given portulaca and honey water to drink. At this point the inflammation spread to the throat and chest – which Rufus seems to have interpreted as the dispersal of the clot of sickness material. He performed blood-letting from the man's tongue, and increased the solvent elements in the compresses applied and the gargles administered, whereupon the infection moved to the knee, and then disappeared.

It may be correct to explain the unusual detail of this therapeutic process as the result of either the prolixity or the unsureness of Rufus, but it seems more plausible to infer from the elaborate procedure he depicts that physicians were moving into increasingly professional modes of treating their patients with more complex techniques. The heightened professionalism of Rufus' period is evident in the diagnostic techniques that he recommends, as well as in the environmental factors which he insists should be investigated. He is explicit in rejecting the approach of Kallimachos – one of those designated as "Methodists" because their diagnoses and prescriptions depended entirely on their preconceived theories, while ignoring the distinctiveness of local circumstances. Rufus insists on the importance of inquiry about local conditions which may affect significantly the disease under observation. Investigation of each specific case is to proceed through interrogation of the patient, taking into account hereditary factors, but also inquiry about the local water supply and determination if there is a pattern of such illnesses as spleen or liver disorders in a certain locale. Also to be asked about are the quality of local produce (especially fruit), reports of epidemics in the region, patterns of childbirth (Questions 13.63 – 73). There is also evidence of the use of painkillers in Rufus' description of treatment for inflammation of the bladder (Ailments of the Kidney and Bladder VII), which includes injecting into the intestines a concoction composed of poppy juice, myrrh, saffron and linseed oil. Specialized surgical instruments are also mentioned by Rufus, including one designed to remove stones from the bladder (XII). To avoid developing such stones, he advises avoidance of water from clay sources and the regular use of filtered water for drinking. Yet in the manner of the earlier herbal tradition, he also recommends trying to dissolve the stones by the use of cold diuretics (celery, cucumber, asparagus, saffron root, and violet leaves, which will cause vomiting) as well as hot diuretics (iris, cummin, balsam, cinnamon). Cold baths are prescribed, but hot baths are to be avoided (XIII).

At the same time, there is evident in Rufus' writings a willingness to acknowledge the severe limits of the profession, as we have already noted above in connection with his description of the inflammation of the throat as impossible to cure. In Case XX of the *Journal*, in which a man is suffering from angina, the use of a compress was stopped, "because an aggressive compress in this situation cannot drive out the sickness material, since it is so deeply imbedded, and because a solvent compress cannot dissolve it. The aggressive means drove the inflammation in more deeply, and the solvent means released it into his body from his [throat]". In this case, the physician – not Rufus – continued bloodletting, which resulted in the patient's fainting, and soon his death. Even though by modern medical insights it would be said that the doctor bled the patient to death, it is significant that by the middle of the second century the best informed of the medical experts were acknowledging the limits of their methods and skills.

To a degree not evident in earlier medical writings, Rufus manifests awareness of what we would call the psychological aspects of illness. In the essay *Concerning the Interrogation of the Sick* Rufus urges doctors to ask their patients not only about such obviously health-related matters as their habits in eating, their favourite foods, their patterns of defecation, but also their previous experience with doctors, and about how they have responded to illness in the past. Did they groan or cry out? What was the position and colour of the body of the stricken person? What was the nature of their hand-grip? Was there loss of speech? How did the patient accept his or her predicament? If it was accepted bravely, that is a hopeful sign for recovery. In his treatise on the treatment of certain venereal diseases,[50] Rufus counsels how to repress sexual urges: take rue; lie on the back, rather than the side, since that position excites erotic dreams; avoid conversation or thinking about sex; eating honeysuckle seeds will suppress erotic dreams; do exercises that will draw energies into the upper part of the body and away from the genitalia; chill the loins with flea-bane and fine meal; if the disease worsens, use cups to withdraw the sickness material; avoid all sexual excitation. Clearly therapy is not viewed by Rufus as a matter of purely physical or even organic concern. Rather, illness must be analysed and treated along lines which might today be characterized as a combination of psychological and medical illness.

Rufus' mixture of approaches to healing is evident in the case histories which are included in his *Journal of the Sick*. The complete contents of one of these is the following:

> The story of another melancholia patient: I know another man who each spring experienced a pain between his ribs,

though it occurred without fever or flatulence, but with sharp pains and tingling. Because of this, he underwent each year a blood-letting and took a purgative. The sickness would regularly last from the time of the equinox until the spring temperature rose. Then the sickness would ease off, after it had been weakened through the blood-letting and the purging. Since he believed that he had not really been helped by these two types of treatment, he gave them up. Indeed, the pain, which lasted a month, was scarcely endurable, and even mounted into his chest. So once again he had the blood-letting performed and took the purgative. The pain did not ease off, however, but spread to the region of his face, where he could feel it on one side. Then after·a time it settled in his jawbone. Since I now feared that it would reach his eyes and brain, I ordered him to have a blood-letting and three times to take a purgative. Also I cauterized the painful spot between his ribs, since it was there that the pain was most concentrated.

For days he had nothing to complain about, but on the fifth day, he began to see phantoms before his eyes. I would not risk another purge because his body was already so dried out. So I prescribed for him moist diet with which the evacuation could be achieved, if I had to resort to that. The phantoms remained two days; on the third he showed symptoms of melancholy. Then he abandoned hope. None of his symptoms dismayed me, however, since I had become convinced that I had already gotten rid of the sickness material. Then I nourished him for about thirty days with barley juice, with rock-fish and with soup made of horse-bones. The more moist his body became, the more the symptoms of melancholy faded away, until he was completely healed.

The symptoms of melancholy which afflicted him consisted of worry and fear at the prospect of death. For this reason I ordered him to engage in play and pastimes. After eighty days, he had recovered. The doctors could not explain how he had gotten better; that is, how the sickness material had shifted after the purging to a nobler part of his body and how the sickness had gone away from him without a further purgation. Then I showed them that there had been enclosed in his arteries a waste-deposit of black bile. It had continually corrupted and damaged the blood in his arteries. After we had emptied it out, a bit of it still remained. But because we had removed the basic cause, its effects kept diminishing. When it finally reached his brain, he had already become extremely weak, and there were still in him dry, scalded fluids which had manifested themselves in the patient in the form of his worry and sleeplessness. Consequently, the remnants of them became a catalyst for more fluids, which were converted into black bile and produced melancholy. After we prescribed for him a moist diet and allayed his anxieties, the disease disappeared.[51]

The influence of philosophical tradition is also evident in Rufus' writings. Serving as a bridge from his essay *On the Names of the Parts of the Body* to the one *On the Anatomy of Parts of the Body*,[52] is a passage in which the place of human beings within the cosmic order is addressed: "Man in effect, in the eyes of philosophers, is a microcosm; he is the representation of the beautiful order of heavenly things, manifesting an art varied as to the construction of the parts and as to the achievement of their functions. Consequently it is important to learn the subjects of study which anatomy as well as other branches of medicine supply. Posing the principles of art as fundamental for our instruction, we declare what place Nature assigns to each part and what name she imposes on each." One may see in this philosophical statement traces of the Platonic notion of the heavenly archetypes, of the Stoic belief in natural law, with hints of the biblical notion from Genesis of the divine naming of the earthly creatures. The atmosphere of these lines is that of a reverent philosopher, not that of a relentlessly rationalistic scientist who excludes from his thinking all but the data presented by his sensory experience. That perspective becomes even more explicit in Galen, who stands as the greatest of the medical figures – not only from the period of our specific concern, but from the late classical world as a whole.

8. Galen

In his brilliant study, *Greek Sophists in the Roman World*, G. W. Bowersock observes that in the later second century A.D. "Galen acquired an eminence and prestige among the aristocrats of Rome such as no doctor before him".[53] Over the centuries the social standing of physicians had waxed and waned. In the fifth century B.C.

there had been an unusual collocation of genius at a time when
Socrates, Euripides, Thucydides, and Hippocrates were simultaneously active in Greece. And as Bowersock notes, "the abundance,
professionalism, and social standing of physicians seem often to vary
in direct proportion to the refinement of the culture ..."[54] It was
precisely "during the flowering of the so-called Second Sophistic
movement" that Galen emerged as the leading figure in the realm of
medicine, or that, analogous to the fifth-century B.C. "nexus between
philosophy, oratory and medicine", his period of prominence "was
accompanied by a wave of popular enthusiasm for medicine".[55] The
advances in medical insight had largely been made in earlier centuries,
but Galen was both the leader and the beneficiary of the convergence
of factors in the Second Sophistic period.

Both his output and the range of his learning were enormous. It
has been estimated that in modern published form his works would
fill twelve volumes of 1,000 pages each. The scope and quality of his
learning are evident in such fields as mammalian gross morphology,
dissection, and pharmacology, as well as through his commentaries
on Hippocrates and his observations about Plato, Aristotle, the Stoics
and principles of logic. Born under Hadrian (ca 130), he died about
200, under Septimius Severus, thereby effectively spanning the
brilliant Antonine epoch. Galen's studies in Pergamum, Smyrna and
Corinth helped prepare him for his career, but especially important
was his stay in Alexandria, where the availability of human bones for
the study of anatomy made a major contribution to his information
about the human body and his outlook on medicine. As Owsei Temkin
has noted, the influence of Aristotle is apparent in Galen's acceptance
of the doctrine of four elements, and that of Plato is to be traced in
his view of truth and beauty, whereby perception is the criterion of
sensible things, and intelligence that of intelligible things.[56]

As we noted earlier concerning the post-Enlightenment attempt to
portray the Hippocratic tradition as the forerunner of modern scientific rationalism, there is a kindred desire in some quarters to portray
Galen as the prototype of the rationalistic, scientific humanist. What
has been said about the Enlightenment's adulation of Hippocrates
as the epitome of reason is equally suitable for the exaltation of Galen:
in the Enlightenment the enemies of truth are "priests, tyrants, and
philosophical speculation, whereas progress comes from the unique
genius, who puts his mind to nature as it is commonly observed by
all".[57] That evaluation is evident in the statement by L. G. Ballester
that, "The new feature in Galen is the insistence that scientific

diagnosis be made solely on the basis of reason ... Observations should produce not a mere opinion (δόξα), but knowledge based on evidence (ἐπιστήμη σαφής). He operated, we are told, "on the Aristotelian principle of generalization by induction, but his nosology [i.e., his scheme for classification of diseases] rested on his conviction that he knew ultimate reality; his nosography [i.e., his systematic description of diseases], similarly optimistic, was based on his assumptions, rather than wholly on inductive reasoning, as in modern science".[58] Or again, "What Galen called scientific diagnosis (ἐπιστημονική διάγνωσις) is that which unites experience of the senses with functional anatomical knowledge and the exercise of inductive reasoning in the sense that Aristotle gave to this logical process." The evidence on which the induction is based, Ballester writes, includes the clinical signs, together with evidence from the course of the disease, the totality of the patient's organism and habits, the season of the year and the place of residence. "With all this, and of course, basing himself on anatomy and physiology, the doctor will reach coherent conclusions." Having thus constructed his case for the rationality and scientific objectivity of the diagnostic process, Ballester then undermines his case by his assertion that the physician could then make a medical conjecture [sic!] (τεχνικὸς στοχασμός), based on careful recognition of such symptoms as were discernible. On this basis, the argument runs, Galen can convert a conjectural or "indicative" sign, through his diagnostic process, into an "evidential sign" (συλλογιστηκὸν σημεῖον), "thus making the basic structure of a 'scientific' diagnosis possible".[59]

Unfortunately this evaluation – valid as it is within limits – ignores two fundamental aspects of the evidence from Galen. While it is true that the blend of (1) detailed knowledge of anatomy, (2) attention to the condition of the patient, both psychologically and environmentally, and (3) of the attempt at careful theorizing and generalizing, combined to pave the way for both medieval and modern medical practice, the serious flaw in Galen's medical system lies in his assumptions about humours and functions of the organs of the body. But further, Galen manifests confidence in dreams and in the direct action of Asklepios which cannot be reduced to what Ballester means by "evidential signs". After surveying some of the important insights of Galen in anatomy and physiology, we shall examine some of the religious factors which Galen regarded as harmonious with his medical research and practice.

In contrast to earlier Greek medicine, in which the method was based on a combination of personal observation and theories about humours (Hippocrates), Galen further refined the late Hellenistic and earlier Roman emphasis on anatomy as basic. In his work *On Anatomical Procedures*,[60] he reports how by coming upon some human skeletons that had been exposed, he was able to learn anatomy at first hand and in detail, and how he supplemented this by the study of apes (I.2–3). This knowledge had been useful for, and was also supplemented by, his work with those wounded in warfare. In the course of extracting missiles, excising bones, and treating dislocations, one must have accurate knowledge of all parts of the arms and legs, of the internal and external parts of the shoulders, the back, the ribs, the abdomen, and the head, "For it is from these that we have to extract weapons, incising the contiguous areas, excising some parts, evacuating humours in putrid infections and abcesses, and treating ulcers" (II.33). He warns that ignorance of these details makes the physician "more likely to maim his patients, or to destroy rather than save life". He counsels that the young student of medicine should learn about the outer muscles and bones before turning to the inner organs (II.3), and warns that unless the physician is thoroughly acquainted with the nerves of each muscle and especially of those nerves which have important functions, the "slapdash practitioner" may slash away, destroying nerves, leaving limbs useless (III.9), or doing permanent damage through attempted surgery of the face and head (IV.1).

In his treatise *On Medical Experience* Galen[61] adopts the opinion "held by the most skilful and wisest physicians and the best philosophers of the past ... that the art of healing was originally invented and discovered by the *logos*: ἀναλογισμός, which reaches a conclusion by pointing to invisible things, and ἐπιλογισμός, which reaches conclusions by pointing to what is visible. The former method confirms prejudices; the latter leads to proper inferences (XXIV). Galen is critical of the dogmatists, who accept as true only what is adduced by *logos* (VIII), but he is also critical of the empiricists, who rely solely on commonsense explanations and cures, refusing to consider theories about or the significance of the invisible parts of the body (XXV). Useful instruments, such as the catheter, were developed on the basis of the visible, and practices such as blood-letting are effective on either dogmatist or empiricist grounds.

In his detailed critical analysis of Galen's understanding of blood flow and respiration, E. E. Siegel shows not merely what the mistakes were in Galen's physiology, but also how close he came to what would now be regarded as correct understandings.[62] Galen understood that the lungs were instrumental in the body's absorption of air, but thought that the rhythmical contractions and expansions of the thorax were the cause of the flow of blood into the left ventricle of the heart, which was the seat of both the motive and combustive processes of the body.[63] He perceived neither the hydraulic pump function of the heart, nor the circular nature of the blood flow.[64] Rather, the heart was an organ for the production of heat, which by using inhaled air transferred heat throughout the body. He compared the arteries to the pipes of a Roman hot-air furnace through which the air was propelled by the force of its own spontaneous motion.[65] Although Galen failed to recognize the function of the capillaries, assuming mistakenly that air and drugs could enter the bloodstream through the skin and that through sweat the expulsion of invisible vapours was achieved, his theories laid the foundation for the anatomical study of the blood supply of the central nervous system. Similarly, although he came close to recognizing the sources of the cerebro-spinal fluid, he had a deductive theory of the *pneuma*, according to which it rose through the brain and escaped through the suture of the bone and the skin.[66] He differentiated two types of *pneuma*: (1) *pneuma zotilon*, which was carried by the arterial blood from the left heart to all the organs; (2) *pneuma psychikon* which permeated only the brain and the nervous system as the specific carrier of nervous and mental activity.[67] Failure to recognize what is obvious to the modern mind – that the common feature in Galen's theory of *pneuma* is oxygen – led to incorrect understanding of both respiratory and nervous systems.

On matters of internal disease, Galen's doctrine of humours was only slightly different from that of his predecessors in the medical arts. He sought to distinguish two types of disease: those resulting from dissolution of unity, and those arising from δυσκρασία, by which he meant (as Rufus of Ephesus did) a disturbance of the balance of the humours. The two types of fevers which these disorders produced were generalized (caused by the decomposing of the humours: phlegmatic, melancholic, picrophilic) and localized (caused by impaction of the fever in a particular part of the body, with resultant putrefaction of the humour and noxious fever).[68] Arguing deductively from this theory of the humours, which went back to Pythagoras and Hippocrates, Galen offered analyses of every sort of bodily disorder, from heart problems, through pneumonia, to cancer, carbuncles, leprosy, elephantiasis and strokes.[69]

In two areas, however, Galen seems to have had some distinctive ideas of his own. With regard to diseases of the blood – which he regarded as the best and most beneficial humour – he assigned circulatory disorders to over-activity of the blood or over-concentration of it in such a way as to cause the hardening of the arteries. Conversely, anaemia was the result of dilution of the blood.[70] His notion of *sympathy* assumed that, in addition to the direct effect of imbalance of the humours, a part of the body could be affected adversely by sympathy with an impaction of the humours elsewhere. This difficulty manifested itself in a variety of forms: (1) through nerve conduction, which produced a stroke; (2) through inhibition of nerve conduction, which also caused a stroke; (3) through transfer of a humour, which produced convulsions, epileptic stupor, or melancholy; (4) through vapours, especially melancholic vapours which penetrated the brain; (5) by direct contact, as when lymph-nodes swelled following the healing of an ulcer. Siegel is of the opinion that Galen made an enduring contribution to medicine by this concept, even though the terminology and the explanation of the phenomenon have changed.[71]

How did Galen, the focus and fountainhead of so much medical learning, see himself in relation to religion and magic? There is a story that when Galen was sixteen, his father had a dream in which he was instructed to apprentice his son to an official connected with the Asklepion in Pergamum.[72] His training was not that of a mystagogue, of the type that prepared people for incubation in the shrine of Asklepios, as they sought miraculous healing, but that of a physician, steeped in the tradition and practices of the medical art. As Bowersock notes, the cult of Asklepios had been in existence for many centuries, with temples in his honour erected in various parts of the empire, and some going back into remote antiquity. In the second century, however, the god enjoyed a tremendous resurgence in popular interest and acclaim. The links between the god's role as patron of physicians and as divine saviour of the ailing seeker were clearly evident, and assumed institutional form in places like Cos and Pergamum where shrines and medical schools were operated under Asklepios' beneficent care. Rational and spiritual healing co-existed.[73] Galen himself credited Asklepios with having saved him from a near fatal disease, which benefaction led him to decide to become a servant of the god.[74] Thus Galen saw his life as combining the benefits of mystical association with Asklepios and immersion in the learned tradition of medicine that centred around the name of the god. It is fitting, therefore, that his essay on anatomy, *De usu partium*, was written as a hymn to the god, in which he expressed his devotion through medical science rather than through the traditional offerings (III.10).

Yet for Galen, even Asklepios worked within limits imposed by the order of Nature. Although he uses the imagery of Greek mythology, Galen acknowledges that the god cannot triumph over the weakness of a sixty-year old body.[75] Just as Nature arranges the *kosmos* in a manner that is worthy of human praise, so Asklepios arranges the welfare of humans in the best possible manner, though always within the limits imposed by matter. The rational order of the world, and especially of the human body, attests the wisdom, providence, power and goodness of Nature. This superior intelligence must come from the heavenly order of things, which is composed of substance superior to that of the earth. Humans share rationality with the gods, but they are corrupted by passion and concupiscence. Yet each should seek to live by rationality, to acquire philosophical understanding, and thereby to acquire the greatest of the good things that the gods have to offer.[76] The chief interpreter of the gods for Galen is Hermes, who is the master of reason and the universal artist as well as the divine messenger. But Galen also considers as "divine" such figures of the past as Socrates, Homer, Plato, and of course, Hippocrates.[77]

Did the gods, and particularly Asklepios, communicate with Galen in matters of detail of his medical career? Did Galen give credence to, or even rely upon the miracles that are reported to have occurred in the shrines of Asklepios? Galen gives a clear and affirmative answer to the first of these questions. His dreams often concerned medical matters, but in spite of the accusations of his critics that he received information through dreams, it seems more likely that he regarded these dream communications as confirmation of insights he had gained through his combination of reason and experience.[78] He does, however, note that some specific medical wisdom came to him through dreams – concerning surgery on the arteries and about a remedy derived from snakes. But these details must fit into the larger framework of understanding based on reason and experience.[79] The difficulty of the modern interpreter in making a sharp distinction between natural and supernatural knowledge is evident precisely in relation to the medicine from the snake. Rufus of Ephesus, among others, had suggested that certain diseases, which were in themselves incurable, could be cured if the disease were to be changed into one of another order. Rufus claims to have been able to change epilepsy into quartan fever, which was curable. That had been confirmed to him through a dream sent by Asklepios. Galen saw his dream about the snake medicine as serving the same function: divine confirmation of the transformation of a disease.[80]

Less persuasive is the inference that Galen believed in those cures at the shrine that were performed in accord with medical procedures or that the physician sent the patient to the shrine when medical efforts seemed doomed to fail.[81] Certainly there was a basic compatibility between the vision of Asklepios as one who works to heal through science and through direct intervention of the ailing suppliant. The proposal by Chr. Habicht that Galen had an official function in the Asklepios shrine has been rightly rejected, however, on the ground that in the *Asklepios Testimonies* (498, 499) there is a sharp distinction between the functionaries of the shrine and Galen, who is described as a *therapeutes Asklepiou*.[82] Yet in the life of Galen it is evident that Asklepios was regarded as not only a healer, but also a helper in all sorts of human situations. Accordingly, Galen accepted divine assistance in a variety of circumstances, such as Asklepios' veto of his plan to accompany the emperor, Marcus Aurelius, a decision which turned out to have kept the physician from experiencing a shipwreck.[83] Thus Galen was conscious of the hand of Asklepios, guiding his professional development and safeguarding his very life.

There are, however, three ways other specific religious traditions of the early Roman period regarded sickness which are missing from Galen: considering sickness to be the result of divine wrath or judgment; adjudging illness to be evidence of demonic power; linking sickness and magic. The idea that human disease is the consequence of divine wrath does not appear in Greek medicine; Galen mentions it, only to add that few so believe.[84] Similarly rejected is the concept, examined in Chapter 1, which probably originated with the Persians, and which strongly influenced Judaism in the post-exilic period as well as early Christianity, that sickness is the consequence of demonic possession. We shall return to this phenomenon again in Chapter 3 on miracle, but here it will suffice to note that this view, though not espoused by the classical philosophers, by the Stoics and the sceptics, or by the Neo-Platonists,[85] has some kinship to the widespread practice of warding off evil powers by means of certain amulets and protective substances, as claimed by various Roman writers, such as Dioscorides.

As for magic, the traces of magical practices of the homeopathic sort that we noted in Celsus are completely absent from Galen. This is the more surprising, in that, as we shall note below in the chapter on magic, this phenomenon was very much in the ascendancy in the second century, not least among the upper classes. However much we may dissent from Galen's assumptions at certain points, he believed that he was operating within the realm of reason, so that the therapeutic process would produce predictable results. There is in Galen's writings no significant place for magic, with its assumption that secret techniques will force the hidden powers to act in the desired ways, for the good or ill of the intended targets of this coercive activity. Edelstein perhaps overstates the case when he declares, "Every form of magic ... is rejected as useless and wrong."[86] As he elsewhere acknowledges, Galen did believe in those amulets that actually worked.[87] Yet in principle, at least, Galen's healing was based on the divine order of nature rather than on the disruptive, coercive manipulation of unseen forces that is the essence of the magical world view. As part of that belief in the divine order, apparently, Galen believed in astrology, at least in the effect of the moon's location in various constellations on the patterns of diseases on earth.[88] What is clearly evident is that Galen did not regard human destiny as subject to exclusively this-worldly forces.

9. Attitudes toward medicine in the Roman world

An obvious question is: did most of the Roman populace share the exalted view of the medical art propounded by its chief practitioners, and particularly by Galen? Galen is caustic in his denunciation of the money-seeking, routine-bound quacks who "enter the sickroom, bleed the patient, lay on a plaster, and give an enema".[89] Both from epigrams and from non-medical writers of the second century it is evident that the medical profession was regarded as being characteristically greedy and fond of public display. Plutarch, in *The Flatterers*, mocks the smooth bedside manner of the day. Dio Chrysostom describes the efforts of physicians to drum up trade by public lecture-presentations, intended to dazzle hearers and attract patients:

> This sort of recitation ... is a kind of spectacle or parade ...
> like the exhibition of the so-called physicians, who seat them-
> selves conspicuously before us and give us a detailed account
> of the union of joints, the combination and juxtaposition of

bones, and other topics of that sort, such as pores and respirations, and excretions. And the crowd is all agape with admiration and more enchanted than a swarm of children.[90]

In his fine survey, *Roman Medicine*, John Scarborough notes that there were two different classes of physicians serving two different groups of patients. The aristocrats had physicians as servants or as private employees in their own establishments, or had access to them despite their high fees and lofty reputations. There were also many illiterate doctors, quacks, charlatans; exploiters of a gullible and needy public. He remarks that "The intellectuality of Galen fails to pierce the growing gloom of an age gradually turning from rational answers posed by the Greek heritage of questioning to the mystical, all-encompassing solutions of religion."[91] By the second half of the second century, there were many wonder-workers and rhetoricians, of whom Lucian draws satirical sketches in *Alexander the False Prophet* and *The Passing of Peregrinus*. In the first of these essays, as well as in *Lexiphanes* and *The Parliament of the Gods*, the tradition of Asklepios has a highly visible role, but one which amounts to a condescending view of the medical tradition. Alexander plans with skill and effectiveness a public relations coup to coincide with the opening of his oracle: a tiny snake, hidden by him at the site of the oracle in an egg that had been carefully broken and then cemented together, makes a dramatic appearance as the oracular shrine is opened, thus signifying the presence of Asklepios in Alexander's consultation emporium (Alexander, 6–15, 26). In *Lexiphanes*, after listening at length to the boring accumulation of rhetorical clichés and polysyllabic archaisms, Lycinus summons the physician Sosopolis to administer an emetic that rids Lexiphanes of his undigested, rotting verbiage (*Lexiphanes* 21). In *The Parliament of the Gods*, the issue of whether or not Asklepios is to be included among the gods is left undecided, but due acknowledgment is made that he "is a doctor who cures people of their illnesses" (*Parliament* 6; 17). Although we cannot generalize from Lucian's satirical remarks about the healing profession – in both its medical and its mystical aspects – we can safely conclude that neither the medical nor the mystical type of devotee of Asklepios was either beyond criticism or universally esteemed in the later second century.

10. Medicine in the New Testament

In the New Testament there are only seven occurrences of the word *hiatros*, and in only one of these is there a positive estimate of the physician. In Mt 9:12 (= Mk 2:17; Lk 5:31) there is a proverbial expression about the physician's role being to care for the ailing, rather than the well. This is offered in the synoptics as justification for Jesus' attention to the sick, the unclean and the outcasts. In Mk 5:26 (= Lk 8:43), as we noted earlier, the physicians have taken money from the woman with the menstrual flow but have not cured her ailment. Another proverbial expression in Lk 4:23, "Physician, heal yourself!", is a challenge to the one who points out problems that he must cure them. In Col 4:14, Luke is identified as "the beloved physician", with no indication of the nature of the medical role that he may have performed. Those scholars who have tried to show that Paul's companion in the narratives of Acts was the physician, Luke, have not only failed to make their case,[92] but are unable to explain why it is that, when (*ex hypothesi*) Paul is bitten by a poisonous viper, his medical companion seemingly makes no move to assist him, nor does he try to cure the father of Protos (Acts 28). It seems clear that the author of Acts does not look to physicians for cures, but to God who acts directly on behalf of needy, seeking persons. But this brings us to the next theme to which we shall turn our attention: miracle.

Before doing so, however, some observations may be in order about the relation of medical technique to healing in the gospel narratives. We shall examine in the next chapter the claims of the form critics, who have sought to show parallels between the healing stories of the gospel tradition and those of the Hellenistic tradition, and who have assumed that the therapeutic methods of the Graeco-Roman medical tradition have influenced the ways in which the healings attributed to Jesus are reported.[93] Ironically, nearly all the evidence used by the form critics is unsuitable because the alleged parallel material dates from the mid- to late second or early third century, and is therefore scarcely appropriate as a prototype for the gospel tradition. As we shall see in the chapter on miracle, there are earlier Jewish and Graeco-Roman materials which are more nearly analogous to the gospel healing accounts than those adduced by the form critics, but these describe the direct actions of divine beings – particularly Asklepios and Isis – rather than healings performed by humans. But with regard to any influence on the gospels from ancient medical technique, there is in the gospels not a single instance of the technical language or methods of the medical tradition from the time of Hippocrates to Galen – nothing of humours, *dyskrasia*, or any of the distinctive therapies of the medical tradition. The two seeming exceptions are the instruction by Jesus to the leper to make arrangements for being cleansed in the temple (Mk 1:44; Lk 5:14) and to the man born blind to wash in the pool of Siloam (Jn 9:1–41). But in both cases what is at stake is not the drawing out of a humour or a "sickness material", such as we might find in Celsus. Rather the issue is very different, involving a factor of dominant significance in a movement that took its rise within Judaism: it is one of ceremonial purity, in order to qualify for participation in the covenant community. This is explicit in Jesus' reported response: "Offer for your cleansing what Moses commanded, for a proof to the people." Similarly in John 9, the religious leaders cannot accept Jesus' healing of the man born blind, because the washing took place at Jesus' instruction in violation of the sabbath law, and therefore of the integrity of the covenant people. The superficial similarity of some of the healing techniques used by Jesus to those used in Greece and Rome should not lead one to overlook the fundamentally different frameworks of meaning in which they stand.

3

MIRACLE

There is abundant evidence from the Hellenistic and early Roman periods for the flourishing of healing shrines and for the belief in the direct intervention of the gods for healing purposes – the phenomenon we have defined as miracle. Alongside this is the evidence for the developing medical tradition which we surveyed in the previous chapter. From literary, inscriptional and archaeological sources comes extensive information about the miracle-working gods and goddesses of the first two centuries of our era. Chief among these wonder-working divinities are Isis and Asklepios in the Hellenistic and Roman traditions, and the God of Israel in the Judaeo-Christian traditions. Although there are discernible patterns or modes in which the divine actions are perceived, not only is there no simple uniformity within any one of these traditions, but each of these types of miracle phenomenon can be seen to change and adapt with the changing context in which it is said to have occurred.

1. Isis and Asklepios

Among the best-attested of the cults in which the divinity acts on behalf of seeking devotees is that of Isis.[1] By Hellenistic times Isis had taken over from Ma'at the tasks of ordering the universe and preserving justice, but in addition she also had come to be viewed as the benefactress of those in particular need who sought her aid. The hymn-like utterances in praise of her beneficent powers (ἀρεταλογία) go back as early as the second century B.C. A text found in recent times at the site of Maroneia in Greece was commissioned by a devotee of Isis who was going blind, but whose sight was restored through the grace of Isis. This testimony is followed by praise to Isis and her consort, Sarapis, who provide health (ἰατρική) to those in need and who maintain the order of the universe.[2] Diodorus Siculus describes Isis as the one who discovered health-giving drugs and was skilled in

67

the science of healing, and who now "finds her greatest delight in the healing of mankind" and in giving "aid in their sleep to those who call upon her". In these nocturnal self-disclosures, Isis manifests her very presence (ἐπιφανεία) and her beneficence (εὐεργετικόν) toward those who come to her seeking aid.[3]

The shrines of Isis were found not only in the major cities of the eastern Mediterranean, but also in the vicinity of Rome, and elsewhere in western Europe and the British Isles. Diodorus is not exaggerating when he writes that she is honoured by the whole inhabited world (οἰκουμένη) for her revealing of herself and her powers to those in need:

> For standing above the sick in their sleep she gives aid for their diseases and works remarkable cures upon such as submit themselves to her; and many who have been despaired of by their physicians because of the difficult nature of their malady are restored to health by her, while numbers who have altogether lost the use of their eyes or of some other part of the body, whenever they turn for help to this goddess are restored to their previous condition.[4]

The physicians are mentioned by Diodorus only to contrast their limitations with the unlimited power of Isis to act directly on behalf of the sick or disabled. The reference to nocturnal visits by, and the epiphany of the goddess is accompanied by no hint of healing technique; indeed, her healings are said to occur in cases where the medical methods have failed. In the Isis aretalogies there is also missing any discussion of the cause of the ailments; that is, there is nothing corresponding to the analysis of the compacted humours or the presence of sickness material. The illness is simply a given. The goddess acts to restore health.

Although as we have noted earlier, Asklepios is the patron and prototype of physicians, he also functions in the late Hellenistic and early Roman periods in a manner nearly identical with that of Isis: appearing in the night to ailing devotees, healing and restoring them by direct divine action. The experience of nocturnal visitations in the Asklepios cult can be traced back as early as Aristophanes (450–388 B.C.), whose mocking comedy, *Plutus*, includes an account of a visit to a shrine of Asklepios. On that occasion the seekers bedded down for the night in the shrine, disturbed only by the priest helping himself to the food that had been left on the altar as an offering to the god, and by one of the chief characters breaking wind as the god approached. But approach he did, and in one case acted like a physician, by placing a plaster on the eyes of a man with bad eyesight. The other patient, for whom the play is named, was visited in the night by the sacred serpents, who were thought to embody the healing god. The snakes licked Plutus' eyelids, effecting an immediate cure. At this point both the god and his sacred serpents disappeared into the inner courts of the shrine.[5]

Livy[6] and Ovid[7] both report how the god was brought from the centre of his cult in Epidauros to Rome in the early third century B.C. The god had reassured the council in Epidauros that the move was appropriate, and this was confirmed by a serpent from the shrine there that not only mounted the ship carrying Asklepios' image, but also kept watching as it sailed up the Tiber in order to give clear indications where the new shrine was to be located: on the island in the Tiber. The shrine at Epidauros continued to function after the removal to Rome, however, on down into the later Roman period. From the architectural remains and especially from testimonies carved on plaques affixed to the walls of the shrine it is possible to reconstruct both the cult practice itself and the effects that it had on the devotees. The description provided by the second-century A.D. writer and tour-guide, Pausanias, matches well with the archaeological and inscriptional remains.

The sacred grove that surrounded the shrine at Epidauros was marked off so that its sanctity could be preserved: no birth or death could take place there. The image of the god, carved from ivory and gold, included a serpent wound around his staff and a dog at his feet. Both animals figured in the cult itself, since during the night seekers would be visited by and licked by the dogs or the snakes. The central structure was circular, known as the *tholos*. In addition to the rows of columns were the slabs containing the testimonies to the god's healing powers. In the lower parts of the sanctuary was a triple circuit of walls, penetrated by doors – an arrangement made to provide access for a maximum number of suppliants to the sacred springs which flowed out at this point. Those who came seeking divine aid were required to spend a night in the sanctuary, where they might be visited by the god – either directly in an epiphany or in sacred dreams – or by his surrogates, the sacred snakes and dogs. "It is easy to imagine the vigil of the suppliants, lying in the total darkness of the *abaton*, listening for the padding feet of the priests or the sacred dogs, or the nearly noiseless slithering of the sacred snakes."[8] The visual images were, of course, the epiphany of the god himself, come to heal the wound or solve the problem or meet the need of the devout seeker.

The testimonies from Epidauros follow a clearly defined pattern: the suppliant is identified by name and place of residence; the nature of the ailment or problem is given in summary form; then follows the description of the divine action and the successful outcome. The ailments and disabilities listed in the testimonies include facial and mouth injuries, dumbness, kidney and gall stones, extended pregnancies, leeches, baldness, dropsy, tumours, lice, worms, headaches, infertility, tuberculosis, disfigured limbs, wounds from weapons, and blindness. The problems brought to Asklepios for solution include a broken cup, a lost child, and a lost treasure. Unlike Cos, where the establishment honouring Asklepios has yielded to excavators the remains of an operating theatre, with all sorts of medical apparatus (levers, beams, knives, apothecary equipment), at Epidauros there is no evidence of a medical installation or of the tools of a physician. Neither is there any indication of treatment or ritual performed before or after the incubation in the shrine itself. What happened at this shrine was perceived to be solely the result of the direct action of the god.

2. Jewish Apocalyptic

In the Jewish tradition of the later Hellenistic period there is not only evidence of medical practice resembling that of the wider Graeco-Roman world, as evident in the Qumran document (4Q Therapeia) which we examined in Chapter 2, but there are also claims made for direct divine intervention in human affairs, both individual and corporate. As we noted in Chapter 1, there is a basic feature of the Jewish tradition which differentiates it sharply from that of the Graeco-Roman: much of Judaism had adopted a dualistic worldview, which led it to see human problems — of the individual as well as of the nation — as the result of machinations by superhuman powers opposed to the divine will. This view probably infiltrated Jewish thinking during the time of the exile of Israel in Babylon. The shift from a basically monistic view to the dualistic outlook is apparent in a comparison of two accounts of the story of David's sin in having taken a census of his people: in the pre-exilic account in II Sam 24:1, where Yahweh's anger incites him to have David take the census, thereby intruding on the divine secret as to who the people of God are and what is their destiny. In the post-exilic story of the same incident in I Chron 21:1 it is Satan, the divine Adversary, who motivates David to do this wickedly inappropriate act. Satan appears as the heavenly accuser in Job 1:6 and Zech 3:1. In the apocalyptic tradition, however, what is central is not the title, Satan, or its equivalent, but the conviction that the present world-order is under the control of the God-opposing powers. Both the religious and the political leadership have fallen under the domination of evil. Only those who remain faithful in spite of threats of punishment or even of death will live to see the divine vindication when it takes place in the near future, at a time that God will reveal to the faithful.

In Daniel, the indicators of what God has in store are disclosed to the earthly rulers, who acknowledge the significance of what they have seen take place. As I pointed out elsewhere in an analysis of "The Social and Conceptual Development of Hasidism",[9] in Daniel the pagan kings issue royal decrees in which they point out what God is doing to demonstrate his purpose for his people. Nebuchadnezzar declares, following God's deliverance of the three faithful Jews who refuse under pain of death to worship the golden image set up by royal decree:

> It has seemed good to me to show the signs and wonders
> that the Most High God has wrought toward me.
> How great are his signs, how mighty his wonders!
> His kingdom is an everlasting kingdom,
> and his dominion is from generation to generation.
> (Dan 4:2–3)

Or again in Dan 6:26–7, Darius, on seeing God's deliverance of Daniel from the lion's den, where he had been thrown because of his persistence in defying the imperial decree against praying to anyone other than the king, issues a decree concerning the God of Daniel:

> for he is the living God, enduring forever;
> his kingdom shall never be destroyed,
> and his dominion shall be to the end.
> He delivers and rescues,
> he works signs and wonders, in heaven and on earth,
> he who has saved Daniel from the power of the lions.

What might be called the miracles of divine deliverance of those who remain steadfast in their devotion to and obedience toward God, are designated "signs" and "wonders" in Daniel. Similarly in the

Testaments of the XII Patriarchs, the faithful are vindicated for their steadfastness in the face of diabolical opposition, making war on Beliar, who is represented as being the leader of the hosts of evil (Test Levi 5:10, 6:4, Benj 3:3). Using another image and title, the Dragon is crushed (cf. Psa 74:13) in Test Asher 7:3. In the Genesis Apocryphon from Qumran, the story of the curse that fell on Pharaoh for taking Sarai as his wife is retold in a dualistic framework, according to which Pharaoh is punished for his misdeed by being possessed of a demonic power, which is expelled through exorcism (1Q GA 20). From I Enoch emerges a similar picture: the problems of the present are but a visible side of the cosmic conflict between God and his superhuman adversaries. The fault lies with the lustful angels, who were the cause of the corruption of the human race (I En 6:1–8). Among the evil consequences of the activities of the fallen angels is that they taught human beings "charms and enchantments, and the cutting of roots and made them acquainted with plants" (I En 7:1–6). In short, they gave to humanity instructions in medicine, which is here sketched as a form of magic. In I Enoch 65:10, one of the specific reasons for the condemnation of the wicked angels and humans is their sorceries. Noah, as the representative of the righteous, is advised to hide until the judgments on the earth and its population are passed (I En 10). One of the basic images for the divine renewal of the creation is, in keeping with the Old Testament tradition, healing (I En 10:7). This will manifest itself in the abundance of fruit and productivity of the earth as well as of its inhabitants (I En 10:17–19; 67:3), including the Gentiles (I En 10:21; 48:4). Conversely, the wicked are told that there will be no healing for them, because of their sins (I En 95:4). The outcome is sure, in that God's rule over his creation will ultimately be re-established. Meanwhile, however, the faithful will suffer, but God's assurance of ultimate divine deliverance and vindication is given in the signs and wonders which he is performing for the encouragement of his own people in the presence of his and their adversaries.

A similar point of view is evident in such canonical texts as Isa 26:16–21 and 35:1–10. In the first of these apocalyptic passages, the sufferings of the righteous and their ultimate deliverance are pictured under the image of a woman experiencing the pains of childbirth and the joy of being delivered of the child. Yet the oracle goes beyond the metaphor of gestation to the promise of resurrection: "Thy dead bodies shall live; their bodies shall rise. O dwellers in the dust, awake and sing for joy" (26:19). The imagery of healing is even more explicitly used in the description of the New Exodus and Entry into the Land that is depicted in Isaiah 35. There we have the promise, familiar from its paraphrase in the gospel tradition (Mt 11:5; Lk 7:22) in Jesus' response to the questions from John the Baptist. The geological and geographical renewal of the land (35:1–2, 6b–9) is accompanied by the opening of the eyes of the blind, the recovery of hearing by the deaf, of speech by the dumb. The culmination is the return to the land of "the ransomed of the Lord" (35:10). Healing is not only the symbol, but now also the substance, of God's redemption of his people.

It is precisely in these perspectives that the miracle stories are told in the synoptic Gospels. Jesus' public activity is launched – following his forty days of struggle with Satan (Mk 1:12–13) – with the announcement of the nearness of the kingdom of God. That this implies the defeat of the powers of evil is made explicit in the rhetorical question spoken by the demons on the occasion of Jesus' first miracle (Mk 1:23–6): "What have you to do with us, Jesus of Nazareth? Have you come to destroy us?" This is precisely what he has come to accomplish, as is apparent from his response: the expulsion of the demons. That understanding of Jesus' exorcisms is made explicit in the tradition reported in Lk 11:20 (= Mt 12:28): "If it is by the finger of God that I cast out demons, then the Kingdom of God has come upon you." To the extent that the powers of evil are already being overcome, God's Rule is already manifesting itself in the present.

Some of Jesus' contemporaries put a very different construction on what he was performing, however. The Jewish religious leaders, observing his exorcisms, do not dismiss him as a trickster or as a fake, but infer that he is able to control the demons because he is in league with their leader, whom the religious authorities call Beelzebub, or Beelzebul. In this way they want to consign him to the diabolical forces that Jews thought were at work in their time. One of the reasons for this negative estimate of Jesus' work is that his miracles had sign values in addition to pointing to the defeat of the Adversary and the vindication of the faithful: they also implied a redefinition of who the truly faithful community members were. And they did so in such a way as to challenge the guidelines of community definition[10] that prevailed in Judaism in this period.

Jews were not agreed among themselves as to what was the essence of Jewishness. For some (the Sadducees) it was faithful participation in the temple ritual. For others, it was life as a citizen of a Jewish free state, and therefore their energies were devoted to nationalistic causes. For the Pharisees, who had become disillusioned with the political leadership in the second and first centuries B.C. under the Hasmonean family, the religious tradition was interpreted in terms of their voluntary participation in the informal gatherings in homes where they could read and study their scriptural traditions, celebrating in domestic form the ceremonies that the Law of Moses prescribed for their central sanctuary and observing at the personal level the purity requirements prescribed in Torah for the priests. For the Essenes, who were in despair of both political and religious leadership, the only hope was for withdrawal from society to a place of purity – beside the Dead Sea – where they would maintain their holiness and await God's intervention to defeat their enemies and establish them as his faithful priests in a reconstituted temple in Jerusalem. In every case, however, the goal of Jewish communal integrity was to be achieved by drawing the boundaries of Israel, whether physically or by cultic standards.

In recent decades the work of anthropologists and sociologists has highlighted how central to human existence is the definition of the group with which one shares a history, values, aspirations and basic assumptions. This is as true in the ancient world as in our own time. In the Hellenistic period, aggressive military moves such as those made by Alexander and his successors as well as by the Romans, had resulted in the breakup of tribal units, of regional socio-political units, and the uprooting of long-established cultures, while at the same time these invasions had brought pressure to conform to alien social and cultural schemes. The effect of the Hellenistic and Roman occupation of Palestine on Judaism was profound, as we have sketched above. Sociologically speaking, the question of defining what made a Jew a Jew, what differentiated Jews as the covenant people from the other nations of the world, what special characteristics were essential to distinguish the true people of God from those who claimed membership by virtue of heredity or loosely observed tradition – these were the fundamental issues which shaped Judaism in its diversity, and which at the same time created conflicts among those who claimed to be part of Israel, God's chosen people. We shall see it was in connection with his healings and exorcisms that Jesus most blatantly and publicly defied the emergent Jewish standards of ritual boundaries.

3. Jesus in the gospel tradition

A basic assumption of the early form critical analysis of the gospel miracle stories was that the gospel tradition with its numerous accounts of Jesus' healings and other miracles was developed by the early Christians as they moved out into the Hellenistic world and away from the original Jewish matrix. The aim of the proliferation of miracle stories, it was alleged by the form critics, was to place Jesus in effective competition with the wonder-workers of the Hellenistic culture. To achieve this end, the bearers of the gospel tradition are said to have developed "a certain kind of relationship between the gospel tales and the non-Christian miracle stories, and thus a certain approximation to the literature of 'the world'; not, of course, to fine literature, but to popular literature and indeed to the writing of the people".[11] Dibelius simply asserts that "The miracle is told as an epiphany of the divine on earth, and this epiphany in the miracle is for its own sake." Since tales are too long and too secular to have served as sermon illustrations, they served as proof that the thaumaturge really is a divine being. "This tale-making often, but not always, means a degeneration of the tradition, removing it further from the historical reality ..." and hence is to be characterized as "degeneration".[12] In some cases, it is asserted, these stories were merely expanded from older, simpler forms, or non-Christian motifs were introduced into them, or miracle stories about pagan divinities were transferred to Jesus, thereby putting him "in effective competition with pagan miracle-workers and epiphany figures". In the case of the exorcism of the Gerasene demoniac, for example, Dibelius declares that the story "not only lacks the gospel ethos, but at its conclusion [the injunction not to follow Jesus] is also contrary to the mission of Jesus".[13]

Bultmann makes a similar point in his *History of the Synoptic Tradition*. Some of the miracle stories from the synoptic gospels he attributes to Palestinian tradition, such as the Stilling of the Storm, the Feeding Stories, and the Cleansing of the Leper. But the fact that "miracle stories are almost entirely absent from Q" is to be accounted for, Bultmann declares, not because there is so little narrative of events, but because Jesus is in Q the preacher of repentance and salvation, the teacher of wisdom and the Law, while in Mark "he is a θεῖος ἄνθρωπος; indeed, he is the very Son of God walking on the earth". It is Mark who has placed Jesus in this mythological garb, and who has drawn on Hellenistic tradition for his portrait of Jesus and for the miracle stories which he includes in his portrait of Jesus.[14]

These purely arbitrary and inadequate evaluations of the evidence derive from the prejudices of Protestant intellectuals, reared under the twin influences of liberal theology and the academic theories of the history-of-religions movement of the later nineteenth and early twentieth centuries. Since the miracle tradition is assessed on the basis of simple external similarities to miracles in pagan culture, and since miracle is incompatible with post-Enlightenment intellectual values and learning, it must be dismissed to the periphery of the Christian tradition. Rather than trying to see what distinctive purpose was being served by the evangelist's assigning of the miracle tradition to a central place in the gospels, Dibelius pushes it to the outer fringes, with a mild rebuke for the misguided gospel writers who included this inappropriate material. By showing – as he thought – that this miracle material had been superficially "Christianized", he clearly implies that it is basically non-Christian.[15]

In spite of reservations one may have about the alleged objectivity of Geza Vermes' *Jesus the Jew*,[16] this work serves a useful and important function in pointing out how basic for the gospels' portrayal of Jesus are the miracles, especially those of healing and exorcism,[17] and how well these narratives fit into the pattern of first-century A.D. Jewish experience. The evidence that Vermes adduces from inter-testamental sources is weightier than the rabbinic material on which he relies so heavily, since the latter is regrettably of such uncertain date. But the basic image of Jesus as one among other charismatic healers and exorcists of the time is a welcome antidote to the form critical determination to assign this strand of the tradition to a late Hellenistic stage of redaction.

This coercive handling of evidence could be regarded as the regrettable excess of someone, like Dibelius, who was at the founding stages of a new discipline, form criticism, which was to prove of such value in differentiating the units of the tradition from the frameworks in which the gospel writers have placed them. But, unfortunately, these prejudices are still taken as historically demonstrated evidence by scholars today who likewise want to get rid of the miracle traditions, which they find intellectually and theologically difficult to handle. Rather than trying to analyse the gospel miracle tradition in its own context, taking into account the features which differentiate it from the Hellenistic miracle tradition and which link it to the issues of Jewish purity as reflected in the gospels, they likewise assign it to the misguided propagandizing of later generations of Hellenistic Christians.

The logical and methodological difficulties inherent in this approach to the miracles are serious and require a challenge. The fact that the form critics have made major contributions to their field, and in the process have given evidence of prodigious learning, does not exonerate them from the charge of reductionism in their handling of the New Testament evidence. The prototype for this Procrustean approach to the analysis of historical evidence by German intellectuals is Adolf von Harnack, whose vast learning is evident in his detailed and insightful studies of early Christianity.[18] Yet when he came to setting forth what he called "the essence of Christianity"[19] he reduced the complex array of data to three items which were compatible with the dominant idealist philosophy of Germany at the time: the fatherhood of God, the brotherhood of man, and the infinite worth of the human soul. In addition to the attractive qualities of neatness and succinctness, this epitome of early Christianity has the advantage of intellectual respectability, in that it implicitly brushes off as unimportant or disposable such features of the Christian tradition as apocalyptic, eschatology, miracle, exorcisms, or charismatic manifestations.

The strategy of Bultmann was formally similar to that of Harnack, even though his philosophical predilections lay elsewhere than in Kantian or Hegelian spheres. His own equivalent of Harnack's essence was *Jesus*, which was perhaps more appropriately titled in its English translation, *Jesus and the Word*.[20] There we read that the essence of Jesus is his call to decision, with the result that those who heed his call die to this world and enter in the moment of decision into the life of the age to come. Terms like "die" and "world" and "age to come" are all understood metaphorically to point to the surrender of values which contemporary society and culture cherish, replacing them instead by the attitudes of love, compassion, service which Jesus taught, and which were embodied in his life and his obedience "unto death", in Paul's phrase from Phil 2:9–10. So long as that reading of the gospel tradition is set forth as a modern derivative interpretation, its beauty and potential power can only be admired. But when this abstract construct is presented as being not only the essence of the actual message and career of Jesus but also the norm by which historical judgments are to be reached as to what is central in the gospel tradition and what is peripheral, the method must be recognized for what it is: a reductionistic circular argument. The essence for Bultmann and his followers derives from the skilful use of an appealing philosophical option – existentialism, especially that of Martin Heidegger – and this provides the criteria for, or at least the stated justification for, historical judgments about the development of the gospel tradition. Naturally, such phenomena as miracles, exorcisms, acts of divine intervention in the historical sphere have no importance and hence no place in such an approach to historical reconstruction.

The historical difficulties inherent in this procedure outlined by Dibelius and R. Bultmann, and still followed by their pupils, are many. The evidence adduced for comparison with the gospel narratives dates from a century to a century and a half – or more – after the gospels were written: Lucian, Philostratus, Greek magical papyri. This material from the late classical literature embodies basic shifts in the worldviews prevalent from the first part of the first century A.D. down into the second and third centuries. Evident as those changes are, they are ignored by the interpreters who stand in this older history-of-religions tradition. As is true in the analysis of any historical evidence, it is historically irresponsible to attempt reconstructions of conceptual and literary developments while ignoring the distinctive context out of which the evidence arose. Specifically, one ought not interpret phenomena from the second half of the first century on the basis of evidence from the late second and subsequent centuries, in Roman, Jewish or early Christian contexts. Rather, one must remain open to the range of ways in which miracle was perceived throughout the early centuries of our era.

Not only is it unwarranted to generalize about the healing stories in the gospels on the basis of much later miracle traditions; it is also a distortion of the evidence to try to read into these narratives features of ancient medical techniques, as Dibelius suggests.[21] The centre of interest in these narratives has to do with participation in covenant community, not in medical skills.

Jesus is depicted as performing healings and exorcisms in such a way as to open up participation in the group of his followers in circumstances which directly violated the Jewish (and especially Pharisaic) rules of separation. He performed healings on the sabbath, in defiance of the ancient law against work on the seventh day (Mk 3:1–6). He assumed divine prerogatives in pronouncing the forgiveness of the sin that might have caused the sickness he was healing (Mk 2:1–12). He healed persons who were off-limits by the standards of Jewish piety, by reason of their occupation (a tax-collector; Lk 19:1–10), their race (Mk 7:24–30), their place of residence (Mk 5:1–20, in a tomb in pagan territory), or their ritual condition (Mk 1:40–5, a leper; Mk 5:25–34, a woman with menstrual flow). And he carried on his healing activity outside the land of Israel, apparently mingling freely with non-Jews and allowing them to enjoy the benefits of his therapeutic powers (Mk 7:31–7). Had he carried on these activities in explicit contradiction to, or even differentiation from, the Jewish heritage, he might have raised some hostility, but he could have been simply dismissed as an outsider and a crank. But the gospel tradition reports that he justified what he did by way of healing outsiders and the people on the fringe of Judaism by direct appeal to the Jewish biblical tradition. Quoting a string of phrases from the prophets (Isa 29:18–19; 35:5–6; 61:1), Jesus defends his activities in response to the question of John the Baptist about the source of Jesus' authority (Mt 11:4–5):

> Go and tell John what you have seen and heard: the blind receive their sight, the lame walk, lepers are cleansed, and the deaf hear, the dead are raised up, the poor have good news preached to them.

And then Jesus adds a poignant note, anticipating that the strict moralist and separatist, John, concerned to tighten the demands for participation in the covenant people, will not understand Jesus' sense of boundary-transcending mission, "And blessed is he who takes no offense at me."

Indeed, there is in none of these healing stories any trace of medical techniques, and, of course, not a syllable of the language of diagnosis and prescription for disease which we find in the Roman medical tradition of the first century. As we noted earlier, the only references to baths in this tradition have to do with ritual cleansings, not with therapy. Neither is there anything that can correctly be labelled magic in these materials.[22] The framework of meaning in which these stories of Jesus' healings are told is not one which assumes that the proper formula or the correct technique will produce the desired results. Rather, the healings and exorcisms are placed in a larger structure which sees what is happening as clues and foretastes of a new situation in which the purpose of God will finally be accomplished in the creation and his people will be vindicated and at peace.

4. Rabbinic tradition

In rabbinic Judaism — although the evidence is slim — there seems to have been a belief that a teacher's interpretation of the law could receive divine confirmation by the occurrence of a miracle on demand.[23] That assumption seems to lie behind the demand by Jesus' Jewish critics that he perform a sign in order to demonstrate divine support for his undertaking (Mk 8:11–13; Lk 11:29). Jesus, however, presents himself as the instrument of miracle only in order to meet the needs of the sick and the demon-possessed. He will not act in order to corroborate his own authority. In the Lukan version of this incident, the phrase is added, "No sign will be given, *except the sign of Jonah*." Jonah's story concerns the divine summons to a man to declare God's message among non-Israelites, in the city of Nineveh. What constitutes Jonah's "sign", according to Luke, was not a miracle, but a call to repentance — to which the Ninevites responded in faith (Lk 11:32). Clearly the point is that the message is self-authenticating; miracles are not going to be performed in order to confirm what Jesus is doing. His miracles are enacted in order to meet human need, thereby pointing to the larger, impending reality: the establishment of God's Rule in the world, and the calling together of a new covenant people.

In the late first century and on down into the second century, however, there was a disposition in pagan, Jewish, and Christian circles to regard miracles as confirmation of the divine authority of the individual performer. In Paul Fiebig's basic study, *Die jüdische Wundergeschichten*,[24] only nine tales appear which purport to be from the rabbis before the fall of Jerusalem. In every case, they treat of divine confirmation or protection of the rabbi as interpreter of the Law. The subject matter includes a miraculous supply of rain and bread, healings and an exorcism. The potency of the demonic forces is assumed, but God is in control and will vindicate his own against his enemies.

As we noted above, Geza Vermes has undertaken an analysis of the miracles and exorcisms against the background of rabbinic practice of the first century. His announced goal in this study, *Jesus the Jew*, is a mixture of modesty, impressive learning, and naïveté. The modesty is evident in his statement of the self-imposed limits of his inquiry: "Since it is always an arduous, and often hopeless, task to try to establish the historical value of a synoptic story, the plan here is not to attempt to reconstruct the authentic portrait of Jesus but, more modestly, to find out how the writers of the gospels, echoing primitive tradition, wished him to be known."[25] Few critical scholars would want to take issue with these declared limitations. Yet the earlier stated dual objectives of reading the gospels without preconceived ideas and "with a mind empty of prejudice" seem not only unduly optimistic, but also to be contradicted by the historical judgments which Vermes makes in the detailed analysis which constitutes the major part of his book. For example, the pervasive issue in Mark of conflict between Jesus and the Pharisees over his setting aside by word and act the requirements of ritual purity is dismissed by Vermes on the basis of an alleged pun in the (conjectural) Aramaic original of Mk 7:18–19 and settled by the flat declaration that there was no doctrinal conflict between Jesus and Judaism on kosher laws.[26]

The major focus in Vermes' analysis of the miracles is on healings and exorcisms. Other miracle stories are "numerically insignificant", or must be analysed by setting them "beside other Jewish miracle tales of a similar kind".[27] The claim that Jesus was raised from the dead is to be regarded "even by academic orthodoxy" as resting on *ex eventu* prophecies.[28] Following on a detailed and largely persuasive survey of the changing attitudes toward healing in the biblical and post-biblical literature, Vermes draws attention to the evidence mentioned above (pp. 71–2) of the belief that the techniques of healing were made available to human beings through the fallen angels. He observes, "The exorcist's success was believed to depend on a literal and precise observance of all the prescribed rules and regulations; the correct substances were to be employed possessing the right supernatural properties and the appropriate conjuration uttered." After quite properly referring to these methods as "quasi-magical", Vermes alludes to "contemporary sources" and to the "common occurrences" of this approach to healing, but then offers only two (late) references.[29] The documentation he offers is from the Mishnah and later rabbinic writings (i.e., second to sixth centuries, or later) – scarcely a sure basis for reconstructing attitudes alive within Judaism in the pre-70 period. He links Jesus with "the early Hasidim", whose "charity and loving kindness inspired affection" but whose "miracles made the strongest impact". The chief difficulty with this model for Jesus the healer and exorcist is a lack of firmly datable evidence. From Josephus there is an adequate supply of stories about miracle workers in the period leading up to the Jewish Revolt of 66–70, but these are depicted by him as false prophets, claiming that through them God is re-enacting the signs that prepared the way for Israel's initial take-over of the land in the time of Joshua.[30] But these first-century workers of miracle are neither healers nor Hasidim. Vermes' chief candidate for a rabbinic counterpart to Jesus the miracle-worker is Hanina ben Dosa, who lived prior to A.D. 70. The later rabbinic tradition reports that a poisonous snake that bit him died, that he could effect healing through prayer, even at a distance, that he had a successful contest with the queen of demons, and that God turned rain on and off at his request.[31] Although Vermes notes that Hanina is never quoted in Mishnah or Talmud as an authority on the interpretation of the Torah, the stories that are reported of him have as their aim the heightening of his personal authority, rather than the placing of his message or actions in some larger frame of reference comparable to the Q tradition about exorcisms and the coming of God's rule (Lk 17:20, Mt 12:28).

Vermes' efforts to locate Jesus as a "charismatic"[32] is too general and too uncertain in its dating of allegedly parallel materials to present a convincing or useful historical model. Ironically, the material that Vermes adduces concerning *magic* (drawn particularly from Josephus) is not only surer of date but fits better what Jacob Neusner has described as characteristic of the rabbis of Babylon in the fourth century: "Miracles ... must be divided into two kinds, according to the distinction herein inferred: first, those produced by divine grace elicited through right action; second, those produced by rabbinical power through the Torah. The rabbi's own mastery of the Torah produced power that he could exert independent of heaven, in the form of witchcraft, amulets, blessings, curses, and the like. Rabbinic tradition often makes the point that these were not powers but merits; even the efficacy of prayer depended on additional moral conditions."[33] This description of what in terms of our proposed definition would consist respectively of miracle and magic fits well the depictions of the wonder-working rabbis included in Talmud and Mishnah. They are of service to the student of the New Testament by way of contrast rather than analogy. Nevertheless, Vermes' insistence on the centrality of miracle and exorcism in the gospel tradition is a welcome counterbalance to the dismissal of these features to the periphery that is still to be found in scholarly analysis that uses form critical method uncritically.

We may infer from the limited evidence available, therefore, that the chief function of the rabbinic miracle stories seems to have been God's attestation of the individual rabbi, as to both personal authority and in his understanding of the law. When one takes into account the fact that the Mishnah and Talmud began to take shape in the period from the second to the sixth century, it is evident that even this interpretation of the rabbis and their authority is largely a development later than the first century. It does, of course, have a very general precedent in the biblical tradition, where Moses, for example, is given a sign to assure the people of Israel that God has commissioned him (Ex 4), or where Isaiah is given signs to confirm his prophecies to the doubting king, Hezekiah (II Kgs 19–20). This tradition seems to have exercised little influence on the first generation of Christians, however.

5. Roman historians

Yet miracle as evidence of divine approbation does appear in the Roman tradition in the time just before the designation of Vespasian as emperor (A.D. 69). The growing popularity of the Isis cult is apparent from the effort of Caligula (37–41) to buttress his claim to absolute autocracy on the Egyptian model by erecting a shrine to Isis on the Campus Martius. The Flavians came to power and were able to sustain their dynasty in part by exploiting the popularity of the Isis tradition. Vespasian was able to make a successful bid for power at the end of the year of the four emperors (68–69) by skilfully sending back to Rome – for popular consumption and in advance of his return – tales of special favours shown him by the Egyptian deities and the special gifts they granted him. Prodigies and portents attended Vespasian's stay in Egypt, including flights of birds, unusual movements of the heavenly bodies and the self-opening of doors.[34] Both Tacitus and Suetonius recount the series of incidents that occurred just before Vespasian left Egypt to return to Rome and assume the imperial power. There had been reports of ancient trees miraculously sprouting on Vespasian's family estate near Rome, but now in the Temple of Sarapis he was presented with sacred boughs and garlands by a man named Basilides, whose sight had been restored, reportedly through the emperor-designate.[35] In Tacitus' version of the story – or versions, since two similar tales are re-counted – Vespasian had had a vision of Basilides while they were eighty miles apart, and from his name it could be inferred that Vespasian was destined to be a ruler. The other report depicts Vespasian moistening the eyes and cheeks of a blind, crippled follower of Sarapis, which resulted in his eyesight being restored.[36] The beneficence of the Egyptian gods – Sarapis and Isis – was thus linked with the accession to power of the one destined to be ruler of Rome. Since the question of royal succession was such an important feature of the Osiris–Isis–Horus tradition, this link with Vespasian helped greatly to lend an aura of divine sanction to the change of dynasties from the Julio-Claudians to the Flavians.

6. Philostratus' *Life of Apollonius*

Miracle as divine confirmation finds its most elaborate expression in the *Life of Apollonius of Tyana* that Philostratus wrote under the patronage of Julia, the wife of Septimius, around the turn of the third century.

One might assume, therefore, that this document and the remarkable figure it portrays are much too late to be of direct relevance to an assessment of the New Testament representations of Jesus as miracle worker. But some scholars continue to justify their use of Apollonius as a model for the analysis of Jesus as he is portrayed in the gospels. They do so on three grounds: (1) Apollonius was a first century historical figure and therefore a rough contemporary of Jesus; (2) much of what Philostratus reports about him is allegedly based on records kept by Damis, Apollonius' travelling companion, on which his biographer has drawn as a primary source; and (3) the figure of the divine man in terms of which Apollonius is pictured was a clear, fixed concept of a miracle worker which continued unchanged throughout the centuries before and after the birth of Jesus.[37]

However, careful studies of the relevant sources have shown persuasively and with impressive documentation that "divine man" was a fluid concept throughout the Hellenistic and Roman periods[38] and can be seen to cover the range of diverse notions which have in common little more than that the individual to whom the term was applied was regarded as having enjoyed a special relationship with the gods. What that relationship was has to be determined by careful analysis of the specific evidence and cannot be inferred from the use of the title, θεῖος ἀνήρ. It is further recognized by most classical scholars that Damis and his travel diary are inventions of Philostratus, created to lend verisimilitude to his narrative, though this scholarly consensus seems not to have deterred New Testament scholars devoted to the concept of divine man from using it as a point of comparison for the study of the figure of Jesus in the gospels. For example, even though the existence of the hypothetical paradigm, divine man, cannot be demonstrated, one New Testament scholar has proposed that Mark's aim in his gospel is to discredit those who are presenting Jesus as θεῖος ἀνήρ by appealing to the theology of the passion.[39] Ironically, what a careful reading of Mark shows is that far from discrediting the miracles as signs of the inbreaking of God's Rule, Jesus is represented as disabusing his followers of wrong inferences that they draw from his miracles (i.e., that they are signs of his accession to kingly, political power).

What is clear is that in the second and third centuries of our era there was considerable popular interest in itinerant wonder-working figures. For this role the shadowy memory of Apollonius provided Philostratus' imagination with a point of departure, just as the miracle tradition of Jesus from the older sources served as a springboard for the pious imaginings of the writers of the apocryphal New Testament. It is even possible that the personal antipathy of the emperor and his wife toward Christianity led to the commissioning of a kind of counter-gospel.

The story of Apollonius' journeys is told, not merely because of the inherent interest in his fantastic ventures and visits to strange lands, but to demonstrate the divine sanction for the life-style adopted by this eclectic, itinerant philosopher. Although he claims to stand in the tradition of Pythagoras,[40] the influence of Stoicism[41] and Cynicism[42] on him are obvious. The reported response to Apollonius by everyone from the king of India to the emperor Vespasian is to acclaim him as a man of divine wisdom.[43] The miraculous gifts which he is said to manifest, such as his innate ability to understand all languages without learning them[44] and to see events occurring at great distances or in the future, are explained as manifestations of wisdom. As he declares to Damis, whom Philostratus represents as his travelling companion, "We have reached men who are unfeignedly wise, for they seem to have the gift of foreknowledge."[45] The gift of divination is the result of the inner presence of Apollo, so that the wise man has the equivalent of the Delphic oracle within himself, and is able to receive and interpret divine communications in the form of dreams.[46]

Although modern scholars have often pointed to Apollonius as the model of a miracle worker, he is depicted by Philostratus as being careful to explain that the cures he effects are the result of either natural therapy or special insight. Thus an ailing, self-indulgent Syrian is cured by a restriction on his diet and his intake of wine.[47] An apparent raising from the dead of a young woman is accounted for by the sage as the result of his recognition of a spark of life within her, which he then rekindles by his words in her ear and his touch on her body.[48] What seems to others to be the display of supernatural capacities in Apollonius is, on the contrary, his attunement to nature[49] and his personal discipline which makes it possible for him to see and understand what the gods are doing.[50] What these extraordinary occurrences attest, therefore, is not his superhuman capacities, but his sensitivity toward the gods and their operations within the natural realm.

There are stories reported about Apollonius' healing skills which sound very much like magic, however. When a woman comes to him on behalf of her demon-possessed daughter, he writes a letter to the demon, who is the ghost of her late husband and who had been outraged because she had quickly remarried following his death.[51] A boy who had been bitten by a dog, which resulted in the transfer of the demon from the dog to the boy, is cured when the dog licks the boy's wounds and then is cured as well.[52] Useful for our purposes is the brief excursus which Philostratus offers on the distinction between miracle and magic. His aim is to protect Apollonius from the charge of practising magic. Magic, he explains, is a matter of technique or the use of a substance or object endowed with special powers for good or ill. When it fails to work, it is to be seen as a result of misuse of proper technique. But further, magicians regularly perform only when a fee has been paid. What Apollonius does, on the other hand, is performed without fee, and is the direct result of his special knowledge of the natural world and of his closeness to the gods. It is this divine wisdom which enables him to expel demons and effect cures.[53]

7. Apocryphal New Testament

In the apocryphal gospels and Acts, miracles are reported as divine confirmations of the authority of Jesus and the apostles. The miraculous actions are about as frequently punitive as they are beneficent, which is intended to have the effect of warning the detractors of Christianity that they may well fall under divine judgment if they oppose the bearers of the Christian message and power. In the Infancy Gospel of Thomas, for example, when Jesus is challenged for having shaped some clay pigeons on the sabbath, he claps his hands and they fly away (2.1–4). When his playmates spoil the pools of water he is making or inadvertently strike him, he denounces them ("insolent, godless dunderhead", 3.2) and makes another companion fall down dead. When he confounds his teacher by uttering a series of incomprehensible questions and allegorical answers (6.1–7.4), his family and the onlookers can only conclude that "he is something great, a god or an angel" (7.4).

In the Acts of John the miracles attributed to the apostle are explicitly said to have been performed for purposes of confirmation of the divine authority of John. Thus the somewhat involved story of the healing of Cleopatra and the restoration to life of Lycomedes (19–25) is said to be taking place "because of the crowd that is present". The aim is clearly to persuade them to the truth of John's message and of the power that stands behind him. Similarly performed for publicity purposes are the healing of the old women (30–7) and the destruction of the Temple of Artemis at Ephesus (37–45), which is done to show that "the God of John is the only one god we know". In the delightful story of the bedbugs who vacate the bed in an inn so that the apostle can get a good night's sleep, and who on the next day are allowed to return to inhabit the bed, it is asserted, "This creature listened to a human voice" (60–61). In the involved account of Drusiana and Callimachus, with its mix of chaste and erotic desires, attempted adultery and necrophilia, the net result is to confirm the authority of John's message (63–86).

Similarly in the Acts of Peter the stories are told to persuade the onlookers – or readers – of the weight of divine authority that is operative through Peter. In the astonishing tale of the temporary removal of the infirmity of Peter's daughter, we are told that it had been imposed because she was too attractive and would lead many astray. Both the curse and its brief withdrawal occurred "to convince your soul and to increase the faith of those who are here" (128–41). On Peter's voyage to Rome, the captain is told in a dream that the ship will be threatened with destruction but will be saved through Peter, so that "of all those who sail with you, let Peter be highest in your esteem" (4–6). In an extended series of incidents which depict Simon Magus and Peter seeking to outdo one another in miraculous, crowd-catching acts, Peter triumphs (9–29). Peter's exploits include a talking dog (9), the restoration of a statue of Caesar that was shattered by an escaping demon (11), and a fish hanging in a shop that Peter temporarily brings back to life (14). The granting to a group of old women the ability to see visions establishes the genuineness of their faith (21). The miracles which accompany the martyrdom of Peter are shown to confirm the divine source of his apostolic authority (30–40).

8. Miracle as symbol: Plutarch and John

Among more sophisticated writers of the second century, miracles are reported as events whose significance is in the realm of the symbolic rather than the merely literal. Again this aspect of healing is evident in both Christian and pagan writings. In the gospel of John the miracles are reported as being vehicles for deeper meaning. That is made more explicit when, following the story of Jesus' appearance to his followers after the resurrection, the evangelist tells the reader, "Now Jesus did many other signs in the presence of the disciples, which are not written in this book, but these are written that you may believe that Jesus is the Christ, the Son of God, and that believing you may have life through his name" (Jn 20:30−1). Only one of the miracle stories in John is identical with those of the synoptics: the Feeding of the Five Thousand. But in contrast to the other gospels, where the writer is content to hint at the comparisons and contrasts between this story and that of the miraculous feeding of Israel in the desert of Sinai under Moses, John makes the comparison explicit (Jn 6:25−58). Jesus does not merely give the bread from heaven: he *is* that bread of life (6:33−5). What he offers does not merely sustain life, as does the manna from the desert, but also promises eternal life in the day of resurrection (6:39−40). The miraculous supplying of physical need or the healings involved have become for John vehicles through which the timeless meaning of Jesus is set forth for faith. In Jn 2:11 we are told that the first of Jesus' "signs" results in the disclosure of his "glory" − a term which recalls the crucial passage in the prologue to John (1:14) which asserts that through the incarnation of the Word of God, "glory as of the unique Son from the Father" has been revealed. Hence what is at stake for John in the miracles of Jesus is not merely the evidences of divine beneficence, or even the inbreaking of the New Age, as in Mark's gospel, but the disclosure of the nature of God.

Two of John's "signs" depict healing: the Lame Man at the Pool (Jn 5) and the Man Born Blind (Jn 9). Each is told for the purpose of its symbolic significance.[54] What is taking place in John is what Suzanne Langer has called "the symbolic transformation of experience", in which words no longer refer merely to objects but to certain concepts, propositions, and situations.[55] These meanings are not private but social, providing persons with meanings which are confirmed by ritual acts.[56] This way of understanding the transformation of human experience has been developed by Robert J.

Lifton, who writes, "We can understand much of human history as
the struggle to achieve, maintain, and reaffirm a collective system of
immortality under constantly changing psychic and material conditions. For modes of immortality to be symbolically viable ... they
must connect with direct, proximate experience as well as provide
patterns of continuity."[57] Man seeks in changing historical and
cultural settings to shape images into a cosmology "which both
absorbs and gives dignity to his ever-present death anxiety ..."[58]
This transformation of symbols in the search for death-transcending
perspectives is evident in both these stories, and is made explicit in
the last of John's signs: the Raising of Lazarus in Jn 11.

The man at the pool of Bethzatha is one of a "multitude of
invalids", all of them waiting − for the most part, in vain − for
healing through the traditional means: the surging waters of the pool.
This man had been there for a lifetime: thirty-eight years (5:5).
He thinks that his ailment could be cured if someone would help him
down into the water at the moment that it is "troubled", a feature
of the story, incidentally, which is reminiscent of magic. What from
the viewpoint of John's gospel is necessary for his transformation,
however, is to hear and respond in faith to the word of Jesus. The
break with tradition is dramatized in that Jesus healed the man on
the sabbath (5:16). Jesus compounds the revolutionary nature of his
actions by pronouncing the forgiveness of the man's sins (5:14), and
by claiming that the authority by which he performed this healing
comes from God, with whom he enjoys a unique relationship. That
point is followed up in the subsequent statement of Jesus (5:19−30)
in which he identifies his works with those of God, claims to be the
agent of divine judgment and the criterion for participating in eternal
life. The man is not merely enabled to overcome his lameness, which
had beset him throughout his life; he is transformed and the transformation has become the symbol of the renewal of life.

The disciples try to understand the plight of the man blind from
birth by assigning moral responsibility for his condition, on the
assumption that sickness is the penalty for sin (Jn 9:1−2). Jesus'
response is that his condition provides the opportunity for a disclosure
of the ultimate redemptive purpose of God, and is not related to
individual moral failure. What is at stake here is not merely literal
sight but the illuminating that comes through the disclosure and
reception of the divine purpose: "I am the light of the world" (9:5).
The washing recalls the medical prescriptions of the period, as does
the anointing of the blind man's eyes with clay and spittle. The

religious leaders seek immediately to discredit Jesus, since he has once more performed healing in violation of the sabbath law (9:13–16). The man states succinctly what is the central point of the story as John tells it: "One thing I know, that though I was blind, now I see" (9:25). That what is at stake is not merely physical vision is clear from the latter half of the story, in which acknowledgment of Jesus leads to one's expulsion from the traditional Jewish community (9:22, 35). The symbolic meaning of the healing is made explicit in Jesus' words, "For judgement [= decision] I came into this world, that those who do not see may see, and that those who see may become blind" (9:39). The Pharisees' rhetorical question, "Are we also blind?" confirms that the imagery of seeing and light are symbolic references to discernment of the divine purpose for humanity as John perceives it.

In the story of Lazarus (Jn 11), Jesus purposely delayed his arrival at Bethany, where Lazarus and his sister resided, in order that he might "waken him out of his sleep" (11:11). Martha rebukes Jesus for his delay, to which Jesus replies, that he *is* the resurrection and the life, and that even those who believe in him, if they die, will live – indeed, never die (11:25–6). Clearly what is in view here is more than merely resuscitation of a corpse. The actual account of Lazarus' being called forth from the tomb where he was dead for four days does more than show the power of Jesus to restore the dead to life; it points to the promise of eternal life, here symbolized by Lazarus' being called forth from the tomb. The implications of this claim are made specific in what follows, in that the religious leaders are made aware that both the temple (which is the place where Israel's God dwells among his people) and the national identity of Israel are to come to an end. And out of those who respond in faith to Jesus will come a new covenant people, a new diaspora: "to gather into one the children of God who are scattered abroad" (11:52). The raising of Lazarus from the dead, like the other healing stories in John, is a symbolic vehicle for conveying the significance of Jesus for human participation in eternal life, and for membership in the new people of God. These stories are not simply additional tradition about Jesus' capacity to perform miracles.

Plutarch, in his *De Iside*, scorns those who take the myth of Isis, Osiris and Horus literally, especially the "infamous tales" about "the dismemberment of Horus and the decapitation of Isis".[59] Indeed he does not want to treat these stories as though they were describing the activities of demigods or *daimones*,[60] or to consider them as allegories of the change of seasons or the patterns of agricultural growth and decline. He scoffs at those who "unwittingly erase and dissipate things divine into winds and streams and sowings and ploughing, developments of the earth and changes of the seasons".[61] Equally unacceptable for him is the theory that these myths are garbled versions of the history of earlier rulers of Egypt, written up by later kings for the entertainment or confusion of the populace, thereby contributing to popular superstition.[62] Instead Plutarch interprets the myth against the background of Platonic cosmology, so that the mythic triad, Isis—Osiris—Horus, is interpreted in the light of Plato's concept of creation as set forth in the *Republic* 546 and the *Timaeus* 50. Osiris symbolizes the relationship between the heavenly and the lower worlds. Although the gods are known by different names among various cultures, they all honour "that one rationality which keeps all things in order and the one Providence which watches over them and the ancillary powers that are set over them all". The result is that "men make use of consecrated symbols that are obscure, but others those that are clearer, in guiding intelligence toward things Divine".[63] By this interpretive system, Isis becomes for Plutarch the symbolic means by which humans may perceive and share in the ineffable beauty of ultimate reality. "With this beauty Isis, as the ancient story declares, is forever enamored and pursues it and consorts with it and fills our earth here with all things fair and good that partake of generation."[64] She it is who reveals the divine mysteries to those who are called, in terms of the myth, the bearers of the sacred vessels or the wearers of the sacred robes, but who in fact carry within their souls the sacred writings about the gods and are clothed in divinely bestowed wisdom. Thus they are prepared to pass on to the other world.[65] Curiously, there is in Plutarch's allegorical reworking of the Isis myth no place for her role in the literal sense of healer. She is, instead, the one who brings the light of the knowledge of reality to those in darkness, and enables the soul to find the fullness of life.

The sharp distinction between literal and symbolic use of the myth is not nearly so clear in the case of Aelius Aristides' understanding of the Asklepios tradition as is that of Plutarch in appropriating the Isis myth. After returning from his initial effort to find acceptance as a rhetorician in Rome, Aristides was transformed through appearances of the gods — of Sarapis in Egypt and of Asklepios in Smyrna. But it was during his extended residence adjacent to the shrine of Asklepios in Pergamum that the influence of this god on his health and on his purpose in life was so profound and pervasive. In the

Sacred Discourses[66] we have a cumulative record of the blended experiences of healing and professional achievement. Aristides' favourite designation for the god is *Soter* (I.2; IV.4), by which he understands the work of the god, not only in restoring his health but in providing him with the sense of destiny and the skills to attain renown in his rhetorical career. But even beyond the discernible benefits of health and career is the conviction of Aristides that Asklepios has been directly revealed to him and has shown him his glorious future in the eternal realm.

There is clear evidence that Aristides knew and participated in the medical techniques which were standard in his time: baths (I.7; II.72; V.29), including those in mud (II.51–72), gargling and purges (V.1–10; IV.5–7). At one point, with characteristic naive immodesty, he notes that the physicians acknowledge the superiority of his medical knowledge to theirs (I.57, 62; II.5, 69; III.8, 16–20). But for Aristides this technical knowledge is only the starting point for the importance of Asklepios in his life. It is as though the ailments of Aristides provide him the welcome opportunity for communion with the divinity. The god's medical instructions were indeed followed (I.4), but the major benefits did not come from the purgations and emetics:

> It was all not only like an initiation into a mystery, since the rituals were all strange and divine, but there was also something marvelous and unaccustomed. For at the same time there was gladness, and joy, and a cheerfulness of spirit and body, and again, as it were, an incredulity if it will ever be possible to see the day when one will see himself free from all such troubles, and in addition a fear that some one of the usual things will again befall and harm one's hopes about the whole. Thus was my state of mind, and my return took place with such great happiness and at the same time anguish.
> (IV.6–7)

He was impatient with those who wanted to converse about the god solely in terms of bodily cures that Asklepios had effected, leaving out of account "those things which at the same time raised my body, strengthened my soul, and increased the glory of my rhetorical career" (V.36). It was through dreams, visions and epiphanies that the god's direction of Aristides' life was communicated, including a vision in which the god identified the rhetorician with himself and attested that his skills were indeed a divine gift (IV.48–57). As a result of these divine visitations, Aristides became enormously effective in rhetoric, attracting and holding the attention of throngs for long periods of time (IV.22–9).

Through dreams and portents Aristides was able to foresee the future and to learn about events taking place at great distances (IV.32–4). On one occasion, with which Aristides was particularly pleased, he was given advance notice by the god of a demanding rhetorical opportunity at Smyrna, and fortified himself by eating well beforehand, which enabled him to spellbind the crowd for hours (V.39). His services were sought by and praised by the emperors (Marcus Aurelius, Antoninus Pius, Lucius Verus), so that they were – according to Aristides – grateful for the privilege of having known a man as gifted by the gods as he (I.46). At the end of his fifth discourse he reports a dream which he had while still a student in Athens, in which he saw himself illuminated by a shaft of heavenly light and ascending ladders which took him into the presence of the gods.

In his treatise, *In Defense of Oratory*,[67] Aristides declares that his own direct knowledge of the gods came to him through illnesses which the medical professionals could neither name nor cure. They deal in the realm of probabilities, generalizing about human sicknesses and conjecturing what is likely to be helpful for recovery. Such knowledge can never be complete or accurate.[68] But his own knowledge has been communicated directly by the god, as has been his rhetorical skill. Neither is regarded by him as a human achievement: both have been conveyed to him through direct communion with the god. If the physicians were to follow his route of access, they would not be so inferior as they are to the god in whose name they carry on their profession.

Whether in its symbolic or its literal mode, whether in the context of response of a healing god to a petitioner or of cosmic conflict in which the divine power is liberating and vindicating the faithful human, whether in a Jewish sectarian setting or in a shrine of a Hellenistic god, miracle is portrayed in the epoch of our study as a response to human petitions and human need. The divine is directly disclosed in human experience as an act of grace or in powerful support of the petitioner and his community. The underlying assumption is that the gods are concerned about human welfare and cosmic order, and that they take direct steps to make certain that what is needed is supplied. In interpreting the element of miracle as it appears in the pages of the New Testament and early Christian literature we must keep in mind the range of possible meaning structures within which miracle in any specific context is to be understood. Similarly, we must take into account not only the cultural context from which the narrative comes, but also the changing cultural climate in which the account was written and in which its intended hearers lived and thought.

4

MAGIC

1. Magic and miracle in Roman sources

Lucius Apuleius, like his mid-second century contemporary, Aelius Aristides, reported an experience of epiphany and mystical transformation, although the divinity in the case of Apuleius was Isis rather than Asklepios. The career to which he devoted his later life was that of a lawyer, but this seems to have been a means of providing money so that he could spend as much time as possible on his major interest: as priest in the shrine of his beloved Isis. While his story in the *Metamorphoses* − which is almost certainly in large part autobiographical − has no significant link with medical tradition, it makes contact at several crucial points with magic. Indeed, the story line is launched with the narrative of Apuleius' dabbling in magic, which results in his being transformed into an ass. The symbolic import of that experience is clear: Apuleius is pictured as a braying, clomping fool, scorned by his contemporaries until he encounters the goddess, who delivers him from his condition, and transforms him into a fully human being, in communion with her and dedicated to her beneficent purpose for the world.[1]

In a later work, the *Apology*,[2] Apuleius develops a defence against the charge brought against him before the Roman authorities that he has been practising magic. The scholarly assumption is that he won his case,[3] but his argument gains its persuasive power through his rhetorical skills, his scornful attacks on his accusers and the range of learning which he displays. The basic issue of his involvement with magic is not directly addressed even in the *Apology*, and of course his participation in magic is clearly implied in the *Metamorphoses*, assuming its autobiographical dimensions. His attraction to magic is beyond doubt. In *Metamorphoses* II.5 he gives a straightforward account of a sorceress: "By breathing out certain words and charms over boughs and stones and other frivolous things, [she] can throw down all the light of the starry heavens into the bottom of hell, and reduce them again to the old chaos." In III.17−18 he dèscribes the equipment employed by a magician, which includes metal plates covered by strange characters, bones of birds of ill omen, bodily members of corpses, nails pulled away from fingers, blood, skulls snatched from wild animals, entrails, well water, cow's milk, honey, meal, hair, and perfumes. The correspondences between this partial list and the means of healing prescribed in the medical tradition − especially in the *Greek Herbal* of Dioscorides − will be evident.

Lucius' own change into an ass, as he tells it in *Metamorphoses* III.21−5 occurs as a result of his association with a sorceress who transformed herself into a bird by rubbing herself with a magical ointment. It is when Lucius uses some of this salve on himself that he is changed into an ass. An enchantress is engaged by a baker's wife to force him to be reconciled with her, or to send some ghost or evil spirit (*certe larva vel aliquo diro numine*) to replace violently her husband's spirit (IX.29). In the Roman tradition of portents, Apuleius reports numerous omens: a hen lays a chicken; the ground opens up; wine boils out of a barrel; a frog leaps from a dog's mouth; a ram swallows the dog (IX.34). The medical arts are represented far less sympathetically, however. The most extended reference to a physician describes one who is bribed by a woman's promise of fifty gold pieces to prescribe poison to be given to her husband, and who is said to have had "many such triumphs as the work of his hands" (X.25). Implicitly, the same charge is here levelled against the physicians which we have seen brought against them by Cato and Pliny: that they perform their work primarily for financial gain rather than to serve human needs. In none of these stories, however, is there more than a passing reference to medical technique, as in the false claim that the bribed physician's potion was "a sacred potion, to the intent that he might purge colour and scour the interior parts of the body" (X.25). The dominant features of Apuleius' narratives are of the sort that deal in coercion and achievement of personal goals − largely destructive and retaliatory − rather than healing. And thus they fall within our working definition of magic.

Apuleius' defence against the charge that he is a magician is powerful in rhetoric, but scarcely relentless in logic. Indeed, a major line of argument in the *Apologia* is to declare that, even if one assumes that he is indeed a sorcerer, it cannot be demonstrated by unassailable evidence that he has performed acts of magic. Although he acknowledges that magic is "a crime in the eyes of the law, and was forbidden in remote antiquity by the Twelve Tables" (*Apology*,

Ch.47), he describes the origins of magic in sympathetic terms, attributing it to men of great wisdom from ancient times. Quoting from Plato (*Alcibiades* 1.21.E), Lucius shows the link between magic and the instruction of young Persian princes, who were instructed by the four Royal Masters, one of whom taught them "the magic of Zoroaster, the son of Oromazes", and Plato added, "This magic is no other than the worship of the gods." Again with reference to the attitude of Plato, Apuleius quotes "magical charms are merely beautiful words" (*Charmides* 157 A), and wonders aloud why he or anyone else should be forbidden to learn this "priestly lore of Zoroaster" (*Apology* Ch. 26).

The specific charges of magic that were brought against Apuleius included his having sought fish to be used for magical ends, his having put a young man under a magical spell, his possession of a magical wooden carved amulet and of a small bundle of magical objects, and his having used love philtres in order to lure a rich widow into marrying him. He responds to each of these accusations in detail. As for fish, he associates himself with the philosophers in the Aristotelian tradition who seek to develop complete classifications of all types of living things, including fish, and with physicians, who prescribe certain types of fish for medicinal purposes. Yet the clue to interest in the supernatural function of the fish is evident in his rhetorical question, "Are augurs to be allowed to explore the livers of victims and may not a philosopher look at them, too, a philosopher who knows that he can draw omens from every animal, that he is the high-priest of every God?" (*Apology*, Ch. 41).

In his defence against having placed a boy under a spell, Apuleius comes finally to the point that the boy was an epileptic, so that his condition was the result of a seizure, not of a spell cast by Apuleius. For the seizure he offers a traditional Graeco-Roman medical explanation: epilepsy is caused by "the overflowing of ... pestilential humour into the head" (Ch.51). Or again, "When the flesh is so melted by the noxious influence of fire as to form a thick and floating humor, this generates a vapor", which when "compressed within the body causes a white and eruptive ferment" (Ch.50). If that humour escapes from the body, "it is dispersed in a manner which is repulsive rather than dangerous". If it comes to the surface of the body, it causes an eczema, but thereafter the person is forever free of epileptic attack. But if it is contained within the body and mingles with black bile, it flows through every vein and floods "the brain with its destructive stream", with the result that "it straightway weakens that royal part of man's spirit which is endowed with the power of reason and is enthroned in the head of man, which is its citadel and its palace'' (Ch. 50). It was this "divine sickness" which was responsible for the condition of the young man, rather than any magical action on the part of Apuleius. This all sounds thoroughly scientific, by the standards of ancient Greek medicine. But Apuleius has acknowledged, with respect to the boy's trance, that it is his "own personal opinion that the human soul, especially when it is young and unsophisticated, may by the allurements of music or the soothing influence of sweet smells be lulled into slumber and banished into oblivion of its surroundings so that, as all consciousness of the body fades from memory, it returns and is reduced to its primal nature, which is truth immortal and divine; and thus, as it were in a kind of slumber, it may predict the future". He then goes on to say that the boy must be "fair and unblemished in body, shrewd of wit and ready of speech, so that a worthy and fair shrine may be provided for the divine indwelling power" which will manifest itself in the divination which occurs (Ch. 43). Thus in the mind of Apuleius, there reside side by side elements of (1) confidence in medical tradition, (2) religious dimensions, which look to the power of the gods to manifest themselves in human experience, and (3) techniques for bringing about these desired results – techniques which closely resemble those of magic.

A comparable appeal by Apuleius to religion in answer to the charge of magic brought against him is evident with regard to the seal and the sacred objects. As for the seal, he claims that it was carved for him on commission. He carries an image of a god with him wherever he goes, and follows the injunctions of Plato in the *Laws* to have what is dedicated to the god made of wood, rather than of a costly material. He chooses not to reveal the name of the god he thus honours (Chs. 64–5). The sacred objects which he treasures have been in his possession since his initiation into the mystery of Asklepios and other gods. Again, he justifies his acts in the form of a rhetorical question: "Can anyone, who has the least remembrance of the nature of religious rites, be surprised that one who has been initiated into so many holy mysteries should preserve at home certain talismans associated with these ceremonies, and should wrap them in a linen cloth, the purest of coverings for holy things?" (Ch. 56).

In reaction to the charge of having used incantations and love philtres to lure the rich widow, Pudentilla, into marrying him, he never raises the question about the possibility that he had not used them nor calls into question the efficacy of love philtres. Instead, he argues that it was Pudentilla's son's idea that she should marry Apuleius, that the marriage had not worked to his monetary advantage, as had been alleged, and that the charge of his having schemed to get her wealth was trumped up by the jealous father-in-law of his late wife's son. The nearest he comes to addressing the basic charge of his having used magical means is to assert that if he were a magician of the sort that his accusers represent him to be – "a magician ... who by communion of speech with the immortal gods has power to do all the marvels he wills, through a strange power of incantation" (*Apology*, Ch. 26) – he wonders why they would not be fearful of attacking someone who possessed such extraordinary powers. It is his opinion that "it is impossible to guard against such a mysterious and divine power". To bring a public accusation against someone whom one believed to possess such powers would be to invite violent retaliation at the hands of the magician. While refusing to admit to possessing such powers, Apuleius nonetheless implies his own belief in their reality and potency (Ch. 26). One is left with the strong impression that Lucius Apuleius, in spite of his earlier unhappy transformation and his ecstatic new birth through Isis,[4] is convinced that magic is to be regarded as a powerful force available in the world, which only his happy relationship with Isis and Fortune render it unnecessary for him to employ.

2. Persian influence and the spread of magic

According to Herodotus,[5] the term "magic" derives from the name of one of the six tribes of the Medes, the *magoi*. They became involved in the dynastic disputes which led to the rise to power of Cyrus and Darius. Of central significance for the *magoi* were their claims to divinatory skills, which centred in the highly symbolic dreams which they experienced. E. M. Butler, in her study *The Myth of the Magus*, advances the hypothesis that their views were either a primitive or a debased form of Zoroastrianism, the basic texts of which (the Gathas) go back to the middle of the second millennium B.C.[6] Fundamentally dualistic, the religion of Zoroaster saw the world as divided into spheres controlled respectively by the powers of light and those of darkness. Both astrology and magic were important as means to gain control over the human and the celestial worlds, in order to assure blessed destiny for human beings through wresting control from the hostile evil powers. To accomplish this end, spells, charms, elaborate ceremonies, alchemy and astrology were used by the *magoi*. The antecedents of this view of the world go back, at least in part, to the culture of ancient Akkad, which saw the powers of earth and heaven in a struggle for control of the earth, the heavens, and the underworld. The instruments for gaining control included exorcisms against the demons which caused sickness, pestilence, plagues and all such evils. The distinctions were sharp and simple: what was good was directly beneficial, and characterized by light; what was evil was dark and harmful to human life. In the process of making and explaining these differences, the *magoi* developed an elaborate system of demonology.[7]

E. M. Butler reports the tradition that the Magians, having lost political power under Xerxes in the later fifth century B.C., found their way to Greece, where they came to be highly esteemed. But A. D. Nock's study of the background of the term *magos*[8] points up the ambiguity of the evidence as to the public estimate of this group, which from the Persian side represents them as a respected, hereditary priestly tribe, while from the Greek side, the designation is equated with *goes* (= quack). Nock argued that the difficulty arose from the imposition by modern scholars of distinctions between magic and religion which are inappropriate for the ancient world. But after denying that any distinction is possible, he offers a definition of magic which is defensible and which does indeed differentiate it from religion:

> What then do the ancients mean by *magia*? Broadly speaking, three things: the profession by private individuals of technical ability enabling them to supply recipes or perform rites to help their clients and damage their clients' enemies; the use by the clients or by others of such proceedings to damage enemies; and ... the religions belonging to aliens on any general ground disapproved.[9]

Nock engages in a series of conjectures about how the Persian priests (i.e., the *magoi*) came to the Aegean area; how they were regarded as strange in act and unintelligible in speech, with the result that *magia* became a common term for exotic practices; how miracle workers in general and Christian miracle workers in particular came to be labelled "magicians".[10] The argument is only partially helpful, however, since it largely ignores precisely those distinctive features of magic to which Nock had already drawn attention. It ignores, for example, the specific charges which were made against Apuelius, as we traced above. The factor of technique to achieve beneficial or baleful ends is the characteristic feature of magic, not merely in modern definition, but in the specifics of Roman attacks, not only against Apuleius, but also against the Christians, as we shall see. What Nock underestimated is that outwardly similar phenomena – such as miracle and magic – must be analysed in terms of the life-world of the reporter and of the community which is being addressed. It is not sufficient to engage in broad generalizations about "the ancient world", as Nock did, in this article, and include in that sweep everything from Herodotus and Plato to Constantine and Constantius.[11]

As anthropological studies have shown, magic is a well-nigh universal phenomenon, and is by no means limited to either of these possible lines of development from Persia to Greece and Rome.[12] A model for the professional magician was provided by the revival in the first century B.C. of Pythagoreanism. Pythagoras is supposed to have travelled to Egypt, Mesopotamia, and India, where he learned the magic of the Magi and the Chaldeans. He was depicted as a great healer who, by using magic and incantations in his cures, could predict the future, and command the weather and the sea. By magic words he could summon an eagle, tame a bear, drive away poisonous snakes, or persuade an ox to stop eating beans.[13] The belief in the potency of numbers, which was attributed to Pythagoras, lent itself to exploitation by the magicians as well.

Although the historical rise of magic in Rome is impossible to trace with any assurance, there has survived an extensive corpus of evidence which demonstrates in detail the forms that magic took in the late Hellenistic and Roman periods. This material has been collected as the Greek magical papyri (PGM).[14] Most of this material is late – fourth or fifth century A.D. But Pliny in his *Natural History* (XXX) states that magic originated in medicine, to which were added astrology and religion in Persia under Zoroaster. He suggests that it was brought to Greece by Asthanes, who accompanied Xerxes to Greece, and from there it spread to Italy, Gaul and Britain. He observes:

> Magic is a thing detestable in itself. Frivolous and lying as it is, it still bears, however, some shadow of truth upon it; though reflected in reality by the practice of those who study the arts of secret poisoning, and not by the pursuits of magic.
>
> (XXX.6)

Yet if we take Pliny at his word on the matter of his reasons for having written the voluminous *Natural History*, we must assume that in practice his attitude was not so negative toward magic as his above-announced principle would imply. After having described "the character of all things growing between heaven and earth", he turned his attention to "the benefits to man that are to be found in man himself". He feels obliged to do this, "especially as life itself becomes a punishment for those who are not free from pains and disease", and he serves notice on his reader that it is his "fixed determination to have less regard for popularity than for benefiting human life". This means that, although his compendium includes "foreign things and even outlandish customs", he has striven "to find views most universally believed". If we take him at his word, then his inclusion of what might appear to modern – or even ancient – readers to be bizarre remedies, especially those attributed by him to the Magi, was for purposes of useful instruction, not merely for titillation of his readers (*Natural History*, Bk XXVIII.1).

One might expect, therefore, that an objective listing of natural remedies would follow such an introduction. Instead, after an expression of understandable revulsion at cannibalistic and other ghoulish practices carried on in the name of medicine – including the drinking of human blood, and the use of skulls and teeth to effect cures of everything from toothaches to ailments in pigs – Pliny launches into a discussion of the power of the spoken human word, of superstitions, and of forms of magical powers (*Nat. Hist.* XXVII.3–6). It is obvious that however much he would like to appear to his readers as a rationalistic man of science, he has a deep and abiding consciousness of unseen, superhuman powers that shape the affairs of human beings and affect their environment. In short, he cannot bring himself to discredit miracles, any more than he can dismiss the magical powers which he sees as inherent in certain substances. He remarks concerning the power of rituals and incantations, "As individuals ... all our wisest men reject belief in them, although as a body the public at all times believes in them unconsciously" (*Nat. Hist.* XXVIII.3).

His own reluctant credulity about omens and in the power of incantations is evident when he observes that "remarkable instances" are on record of prayers having been ruined by the noise of omens or by mistakes, with the result that part of the attendant sacrifice has disappeared or been doubled (*Nat. Hist.* XXVIII.2.11). He acknowledges, therefore, that if the truth of such reports is "once admitted, that the gods answer certain prayers or are moved by any form of words, then the whole question [i.e., of miracles and prodigies] must be answered in the affirmative" (*Nat. Hist.* XXVIII.3.12–13). At this point he proceeds to recount events such as lightning striking down a suppliant who made mistakes in the ritual, and the decision to locate the Temple of Jupiter in Rome as a result of the discovery of a human head on the Tarpeion Hill and the subsequent consultation with a seer. Pliny's conclusion is to assert that the human response to omens, prodigies and curses is determinative of their effects: "Let these instances suffice to show that the power of the omens is really in our control, and that their influence is conditional upon the way we receive each" (XXVIII.4.17). Thus, the recitation of the ritual and the invocations of the deities have decisive results as to what the gods will do. He confesses, "There is indeed nobody who does not fear to be spell-bound by imprecations." In spite of his avowed scorn of the Magi, he regards the incantations and rituals as effective in prevention of fires and acknowledges that he and his contemporaries are "always on the lookout for something big, something adequate to move a god, or rather to impose its will on a divinity" (XXVIII.4.20). These beliefs he believes to be present in the writings of Homer, Theophrastus, and even Cato, whom he quoted in denunciation of the medical profession.

Pliny reports that even Caesar had the habit of repeating a formula of prayer for a safe journey three times before departing, "a thing we know most people do today" (XXVIII.4.21). Generalizing on this phenomenon of the power of words to effect change or ward off trouble, he asks rhetorically why it is the universal custom to greet friends on New Year's Day, to pray so as to ward off the Evil Eye, to wish good health to those who sneeze, or why one pours water under the table when fire is mentioned at a meal. Other popular beliefs and practices which he records but does not challenge are that having one's hair cut on the seventeenth and twenty-ninth of the month prevents it from falling out, and that if farm women rotate spindles as they walk through the fields, the crops will be ruined (XXVIII.5.29). He goes on to describe the extraordinary capacities that certain persons possess, such as a consul from a Cypriot family, whose power over snakes was such that, when thrown into a barrel filled with them, they merely licked him all over; or certain Egyptians, the sound of whose voices causes crocodiles to flee. So great is the antipathy of these people toward poison or disease that for them merely to arrive effects cures. On the other hand, the coming of persons bitten by snakes or dogs makes the wounds of those nearby grow worse (XXVIII.6.31–2).

After recounting these examples of extraordinary power resident in certain human beings, Pliny moves to a series of reports about the beneficial effects of effluences from the human body. These are of special interest, since they describe the healings of diseases which are also mentioned in the gospel accounts, and include mention of details, such as saliva and menstrual flow, which figure in these gospel narratives. He states flatly that "the best of all safeguards against serpents is the saliva of a fasting human being". Other valuable uses of saliva include spitting on epileptics during a seizure, which has the effect of throwing the infection back on them, thereby — by means not explained — assisting a cure. If one has been too presumptuous in dealing with the gods, spitting into one's bosom helps to gain their forgiveness. Spitting into one's hand increases the force of a blow one is about to deliver. Saliva is recommended for treating incipient boils, for leprous sores, for eye diseases, and for pains in the neck, though one must then be careful to apply the spittle to the right knee with the right hand and to the left knee with the left hand. Other benefits of saliva include the claims that spitting into a serpent's mouth will cause it to split open, and that a limb that has lost sensation will regain it if one spits into the bosom of the patient or applies it to the upper eyelids (XXVIII.7.36–9). In addition to his detailed accounts of the beneficial effects of woman's milk, he reports that the saliva of a fasting woman is "powerful medicine" for easing bloodshot and watery eyes, and that efficacy is increased if she has fasted from wine and food on the previous day. Of menstrual flow, "There is no limit to its power" (XXVIII.22).

Employing one of his favourite rhetorical devices — "They say" — to avoid having to take intellectual responsibility concerning a cure or powerful effect that he is about to report, Pliny says that "hailstorms and whirlwinds are driven away if menstrual fluid is exposed to the very flashes of lightning", and that stormy weather on land or sea may be controlled by it. Acknowledging the magical quality of these claims, he nonetheless mentions "without shame" that great damage will be done if this menstrual power is used during an eclipse or the dark of the moon. For example, the man who has intercourse under such circumstances may die as a result. If a menstrual woman walks naked through fields, caterpillars, worms, beetles and other vermin will drop to the ground. Plants with high medicinal value, such as ivy and rue, as well as the crops themselves, will dry up if a menstruating woman passes by at sunrise and touches the plants. A pregnant mare will have a miscarriage if she even sees at a distance a virgin who is menstruating for the first time. Nothing can overcome the effects of the fluid, neither washing nor burning. A woman who touches a smear of the fluid may have a miscarriage as a consequence. On the other hand, Pliny claims, there are those who assert that the flux has beneficial powers – for gout, tumours, erysipelas, boils and runny eyes, tertian and quartan fevers, etc. – even when applied in minute quantities.

An ironic note is added, however, when Pliny, having recounted the good and evil effects of menstrual flow, adds, "... There is nothing I would more willingly believe [than] that if doorposts are merely touched by the menstrual discharge, the tricks of that lying crowd, the Magi, are rendered vain ..." (XXVIII.23.86). There is no mistaking that Pliny is profoundly ambivalent about the efficacy of those human substances to which claims of boon and bane are widely credited. Significantly, there is very little said by Pliny in these passages about the gods, other than the expectation that they can be coerced if the proper formulae are used – which is, of course, a characteristic feature of magic, as we shall see. Just as many of the natural cures of which he writes throughout his *Natural History* correspond in detail to the medical practices of the physicians whom he denounces for their greed, so the reports of marvellous powers inherent in animals and humans sound nearly identical with the claims of the magicians, whom he scorns as charlatans. Although he does not address himself directly to the subject of miracles, the accounts that he gives of the intervention of divine powers resemble miracle stories in other traditions. What little he has to say about the gods directly shows that he is more interested in having them conform to human will by ritual formulae and incantations than in soliciting their aid, as is characteristic in the miracle tradition. The distinctions between folk medicine on the one hand – which is Pliny's forte – and both professional medicine and magic on the other, lie in the view of the reality inherent in each. It is in that structuring of the world, adopted partly consciously and partly unconsciously, that the individual establishes personal identity with the group sharing that perspective.[15]

Another Graeco-Roman tradition linked with magic that appears in Pliny's *Natural History* is that of the power associated with certain types of knots. The so-called Hercules knot was believed in Greek and Roman times to have the power to heal wounds which were bound or bandaged with this type of knot.[16] Pliny informs his readers that it is useful to tie one's girdle with this knot every day. A series of passages in his work mention remedies that involve these magical knots. As a treatment for catarrh and ophthalmia, Pliny reports that "the magicians" recommend that the fingers of the right hand be tied with a linen thread. For sores on the thighs due to riding, they say that the groin should be rubbed with the foam from a horse's mouth, and that three horsehairs in which are tied three knots are to be placed in the sore. To enable someone to recover from quartan fever, a caterpillar is to be wrapped in linen, a thread is to be passed three times around it and tied with three knots. Meanwhile, one is to repeat each time the reason that the process is being carried out. Or one should wrap a nail in wool or a cord from a crucifixion and tie it around the patient's neck. After the patient has been cured, it is to be hidden in a hole where the sun cannot shine upon it. For certain tumours a thread is to be taken from a loom, which is then tied with seven or nine knots; a widow is to be named corresponding to each of the knots, and the thread is then to be attached to the groin. If there are swellings of the groin, the big toe is to be tied to the toe next to it (XXVIII.11).

Clearly Pliny is ambivalent about these healing methods, in that he acknowledges that they may be fraudulent, with the result that "the disappointment is well deserved if they prove to be of no avail" (XXVIII.11.50). But he also notes that "to tie up wounds with the Hercules knot makes the healing wonderfully more rapid" (XXVIII.17). For all of his announced disdain for magic, Pliny is remarkably confident in its potential as a means of healing.

Thus Pliny, an intellectual leader, serves as a witness to the seriousness with which magic was taken in Rome in the first century A.D. As he remarks elsewhere (*Natural History* XXVIII.4–9), "There is no one who is not afraid of becoming the subject of lethal spells." Thus magic may be seen as a phenomenon which pervades all social levels, and is seized upon by those in power or seeking it to force their aims on history, either by moving them into power or by striking down those who currently hold it. As Peter Brown has observed:

> Sorcery is not an unswept corner of odd beliefs, surrounding unsavory practices: the anthropologists have shown that belief in sorcery is an element in the way in which men have frequently attempted to conceptualize their social relationships and to relate themselves to the problem of evil.

The importance of magic in the upper strata of Roman society is evident:

> Accusations against sorcerers occur in precisely those areas and classes which we know to have been the most effectively sheltered from brutal dislocation – the senatorial aristocracy, for instance, and the professors of the great Mediterranean cities. It was in just such stable and well-oriented groups that certain forms of misfortune [e.g., an attempt to sabotage a man's good fortune] were explained by pinning blame on an individual.[17]

And the method of sabotage, as well as of counteracting such an attack, was magic.

3. The magical papyri

In the magical papyri, the efficacy of what is undertaken depends on a series of factors. (1) The recitation of an adequate number of names of divinities as a means of forcing their co-operation; for example, Adonai, Iao, Psyche, Eros (IV:1735–1740); Osiris, Isis, Anubis, cat-faced Re, Selene, Kore (IV.100–115, 155, 2340–1350); Hermes, Zeus, Helios, Iao, Adonai, with explicit references to the Book of Exodus (IV.3030–3040); Logos, Jesus Christ, Holy Spirit, Son of the Father (IV.1235). Thus the repertoire of divine names is ecumenical and extensive. The lateness of much of the material is indicated by the use of biblical, and especially Christian designations for the divine. (2) A second factor making for efficacy in magic is the use of forceful orders in commanding the gods. The regular term is ὀρκίζω; also used are ἀπολάσσω and the more emphatic ἐξορκίζω (IV.252, 275 and especially IV.2566).

The instructions to the magical powers are primarily negative or prophylactic: they are uttered as protection against demons, enemies, or disease. Some, however, are love charms (IV.1390–1495; 296–465; 1496–1595). Although the term σωτηρία occurs, it is rarely specified as connoting either recovery of health or spiritual renewal. Fundamental is the magical technique: there are recipes for magical foods, prescriptions for efficacious rituals, specifications of magical words, and the observance of the proper chronology. PGM XII.136–41 reports god as having 365 names – an obvious reference to the potency of the number of days of the year – a detail repeated in XIII.100. In XIII.79–159 there are nonsense syllables and magic words repeated: seven times χι, three times τιφ, seven times χα; each of the vowels, beginning with α once, ε twice, up to seven times; plus 49 nonsense vowels (XIII.182); expressions spelled one way and then with letters rearranged, such as αεηιουω, εηιουωα, ηιουωαε, ιουωαεη etc. (XIII.905). The coercive force of the texts is apparent in XIII. 788–809:

> Enter my mind and my thoughts for all the time of my life and perform for me all the wishes of my soul.
> For you are I and I am you. Whatever I say must come to be, for I have your name and the sole phylactery in my heart and no fleshy thing will move against me by means of a curse, nor shall any spirit attack me, no demon, no ghost, no evil power of Hades.
> By your name, which I have in my soul and which I invoke, there shall come to be for me in every way good things, good upon good, thoroughly, unconditionally you shall grant me health, salvation, welfare, glory, victory, strength, contentment.
> Cast a veil on the eyes of all who oppose me, male and female, and give me grace in all my activities.

Other papyri are arranged as magical charts to procure a lover (XVIIa) or to enable a daughter to recover from a fever (XXXIII), or to guard against the evil spirit, angels and demons (XVIII a,b). In XII.136–41 there is a threat to the great-powerful demon that if he does not do as bidden, he will be reported to the Most High God and will be hacked in pieces. The message ends with a warning that the petitioner does not want to have to convey his request a second time!

The oldest of the preserved magical papyri, P XX, dates from the first century B.C. and includes the instructions of one Philinna of Thessalonica "concerning headache: Flee, O headache! Be off and hide under the rocks. The wolves flee, the whole-hoofed horses flee, hurrying to escape the blows ..." This stance of peremptory orders is also found in P XVI, which dates from the first century A.D.:

> I adjure you, demon of death, cause to pine away Sarapion out of love for Dioskorus, whom Tikoi bore: burn his heart, let it melt and let his blood dry up through love, longing, and pain over me until Sarapion, whom Pasametra bore, comes to Dioskorus, whom Tikoi bore, and fulfills all my wishes

and loves me ceaselessly until he descends into Hades. I adjure you, demon of death, by Adonai, by Sabaoth [there follows a string of now meaningless letters or names] ...

In the remainder of the document the command to the demon of death is repeated five times, along with slight variations in the instructions about how Sarapion is to fall in love with Dioskorus. The attitude implicit and even explicit in these documents is that the divine powers are subject to human orders, and should be told so in no uncertain terms.

A characteristic feature of the intention of these magical papyri is the request for answers to pressing questions concerning one's future, whether it be a matter of residence, health, or business plans. Thus in P XXX, which dates also from the first century A.D., we read:

> To Sokonnokonneus, the twice-great god. Reveal to me whether I should remain in Bachias. Should I make a request? Reveal this to me! To the most great, powerful god, Soknopaias, By Asklepiades, son of Aneios, Is it not prohibited to me to marry Tapetheus, daughter of Marre and will she not marry another? Show me this and complete [the answer] to this written [question]. To Soknopaios and Sokanpieos, great, great gods: from Statoetis, Son of Apynchis, son of Tesenuphis. Will I be saved from my illness? Give me information about this! To the great gods Soknopaias and Sokonupis. Is it granted to me to start a business for gladiators? Give me information about this!

A similar mix of demand and petition is found in P LXVIII, where Adonai is ordered to "burn the soul of Eutyches, so that he will turn to Ereia ..." The final words are, "Now, immediately, at this hour and on this day!"

One of the concerns expressed in the magical papyri is protection for the mummified bodies of the departed, as in P LIX:

> Mummy of Phtheious Saioneis, son of Sertaesis. You servant of the praiseworthy god, Ablanathanalba. You servant of the beautiful god, Akrammachamarei. You servant of Iao, Sabao, Abrasax, Adonai. You servant of the beautiful gods and the praiseworthy. You beautiful and praiseworthy gods, protect the mummy and body and entire grave of Phtheios the Younger; that is, of Saioness, son of Sentaeis, and beware the ultimate punishment of the thousand-armed goddess, Lady Isis.

As we have seen, in P LIX, a crucial section consists of a string of letters which form no decipherable words. Elaborate arrangements of such seemingly meaningless letters is to be found in a number of these papyri, of which P XXXIII, an amulet against fever, is a representative example. It begins with the following line of Greek letters, which decreases at each end until the scheme ends with the single α at the bottom:

αβλαναθαναβλαναμαχαραμαραχαραμαραχ
βλαναθαναβλαναμαχαραμαραχαραμαρα
λαναθαναβλαναμαχαραμαραχαραμαρ
μαχα
αχ
α

The text which follows reads:

> Unresting Kok Kouk Koul, deliver Thais, daughter of Tauras, from all feverishness of the three-day, four-day, or two-day, or nocturnal variety, because I am the unresting god, as handed down by the fathers. Unresting Kok, Kouk, Koul. Now! Now! Quickly! Quickly!

Some of the papyri are more nearly petitionary in nature, rather than demanding or coercive. In terms of our suggested distinction between magic and religion (pp. 2–4), they are close to the religious type, although they include secret formulae and stylized patterns which, the document informs us, are essential to gaining what is being requested. P XXI, which dates from the second/third centuries, translates as follows:

> Hear me, Lord, to whom belongs the secret inexpressible name; before whom the demons tremble when they hear it, to whom the Sun βααλ βνιχ βααλα ’Αμην πτιδαιου ἀρνεβουατ and the moon ἀσεν[π]εμϕ Θω[ουθ,βαρβαραιωνη ὀσαρμεν ψεχει are the unwearied eyes, shining in the starry eyes of humans; for whom the heaven is the head and the air is the body, the earth is the feet, and the water is the girdle. You are the good demon, who produces good things, who nourishes and increases the entire inhabited earth and the whole world. Yours is the eternal dancing-stage in which your name is established, of which the seven letters correspond to the harmony of the seven vowels [i.e., 4 x 7 vowels],

of which the demons, the Τυχαι and the Μôιραι are the good effluence of the stars, from which we receive wealth, fortune, good length of life and a good burial.

So, Lord of Life, king of the upper and lower regions, you who do not withdraw your justice, you whose names the Muses sing, for whom the standard-bearers are the eight watchers Ἠ, Ω, Χω, Χουχ, Νουν, Ναυνι, Ἀμουν, Ἰο, who possess infallible truth: many bodies shall not gain control over me – those who take action against me – nor shall there oppose me a spirit, a spectre, a demon, an evil. Indeed, your name shall I bear in my heart as a treasure exclusively φιριμνουν ανοχ σολβαι σαναχεσρω .. αρχην σε κοπω ... οαι ... νουσι σιεθω βενουαι

Almost wholly free of both the coercive elements and the secret language of most of the magical papyri is P LXXVII, which reads much like the liturgical formulae of other religions, including Christianity:

> Whenever you want to make an offering, whenever you may want to do so, say this prayer in your thoughts, without ac- tually speaking: I call to you, who sit in the midst of the sown field, who dominate all through your power, before whom even the demons tremble, the mountains are afraid, to whom the angels, sun and moon offer petitions, whose throne is heaven, whose storehouse is the sky and whose footstool is the earth! Holy, holy, everlasting, everlasting, controller of the stars, you who breathe out fire, god shod in gold, reveal!
> And then he will give a revelation in all clarity concerning the thing in question, without making any occasion for fear or trembling or scorn. Follow through this procedure in a pure state, and offer incense at the altar.

Not only are the Christian divine names used in many of the magical papyri, but some seem to have risen in specifically Christian contexts. As might be expected, they show a preference for biblical names and symbols, such as Alpha and Omega (P III), and there are direct quotes from Christian tradition, such as the Lord's Prayer (P IX). There are reflections of the Apostles' Creed (P XIII) and allusions to such orthodox concepts as the Trinity (P XVI), as well as quotations from the Gospel of Matthew (P XVII) and John (P XVIII). But the aim of these formulae is to protect from demons (P X), as the recurrent use of *phylax* shows (P Va; XXI). In P IV each of the string of magical names is significantly arranged to form a cross, and the names themselves are chosen from the gospel tradition. Although there are prayers for health (P IX), the main concern is to ward off evil (P IIa, III), and to protect the house from reptiles or the occurence of harmful events (P II). Mary, the Trinity, John the Baptist, the evangelists, the apostles and the saints are all invoked to guard against evil (P XII). Clearly the line is breaking down between religion and magic, but it is the latter which is the dominant feature in this material, since the purpose of the formulae is to coerce the desired results by means of repeating the appropriate words or acts. What is sought is not to learn the will of the deity, but to shape the deity's will to do the bidding of the one making the demand or to defeat the aims of the evil powers.

4. Pagan–Christian controversy over magic and miracle

Ancient critics of Christianity, as well as some contemporary scholars in their study of early Christianity have tried to show that Jesus used magic in his healing activity. Two studies which portray Jesus as a magician are Morton Smith's *Jesus the Magician*,[18] and John M. Hull's *Hellenistic Magic and the Synoptic Tradition*. The feature of Smith's book that is central for our purposes is the chapter, "The Marks of a Magician", where the primary feature of a magician is declared to be that he works miracles. These are performed by those who claim divinity or who have access to divine power. Not surprisingly, the model that Smith chooses to set forth the typical magician is Apollonius of Tyana as portrayed by Philostratus. Once that picture is sketched, Jesus is compared with it in detail. Mark, we are told, represents Jesus as performing miracles which "are drawn entirely from the magician's repertoire".[19] Although it is acknowledged that magic regularly involves some kind of ritual pronouncement or action, and that there is none reported in connection with Jesus commissioning his followers to perform baptisms, healings and exorcisms in Mark, Smith simply notes that the ritual aspect of the tradition was omitted in the gospel accounts. And further, although each of these actions is said to have parallels in Jewish magic, none are in fact preserved, as Smith acknowledges.[20] In short, we are dependent on the author's pronouncements, rather than on palpable evidence.

The eucharist is perceived by Smith as a magical rite, on analogy with Dionysiac and Isis–Osiris texts from the Demotic Magical

Papyrus. The references to the covenant are said to be secondary; what is primary, according to Smith, is the act whereby "a magician–god gives his own body and blood to a recipient who, by eating it, will be united with him in love".[21] Smith then makes the claim (in italics) that "*These texts are the closest known parallels to the text of the eucharist.*"[22] A careful reading of the text, however, calls into question the appropriateness of this dictum. The document was dated by its editors to the third century A.D. Although they acknowledged that it may include older material, it cannot have served as a model for Paul and the gospel tradition. Its style and especially its agglomeration of material are very similar to the Greek magical papyri of the third and subsequent centuries – an observation which is particularly appropriate for precisely this section which Smith is using to make his case. But most significant is the fact that, contrary to Smith's inference that this ceremony is the basis for attaining mutual love among the followers of a god, it is an obvious instance of an aphrodisiac formula. Both the Osiris–Isis pericope and the ones which follow it are intended to coerce the female object of the male's passion to yield to sexual union. Only by reading the synoptic tradition in the light of the Johannine last supper scene (where there is no eucharist, incidentally) can Smith introduce into his reconstruction the "love one another" motif. Further, he ignores the feature common to the synoptic and Pauline eucharistic passages: the hope of fulfilment of God's purpose in the eschatological kingdom. And of course that motif has its closest parallel, not in a third-century erotic text, but in the appendix to the Scroll of the Rule (Annexe II.18–21), where the community meal and the shared cup are anticipations of the coming of God's Rule.

Smith claims that, by interpreting the gospel traditon in the light of the magical material, he has arrived at a picture of the real historical Jesus: that is, "the following coherent, consistent and credible picture of a magician's career".[23] The spirit that descends on him at baptism is "a common shamanic phenomenon" which enables him to perform exorcisms and healings, and on the basis of which he initiates his inner circle of followers into a magical mystery, which includes heavenly visions and nocturnal ceremonies with the disciples "in scanty costume", and culminating in the meal by which they share in his deity.[24] This reconstruction is achieved by arbitrarily joining texts from John and the synoptics, including material lacking textual authority. Left out of account entirely are the explicit eschatological implications of the "mystery of the kingdom of God" from the beginning to the end of Jesus' ministry. The evidence adduced to make the case is assembled without attention to such questions as date, literary setting, historical development, cultural context. This picture of Jesus is reconstructed on the basis of eclectic personal preferences rather than by careful assessment of historical evidence and responsible method.

John M. Hull's study, *Hellenistic Magic and the Synoptic Tradition* blends miracle and magic into a single complex, which he calls " the magical tradition of miracle".[25] Although he asserts that this connection developed during the Hellenistic period, nearly all his evidence is from the Greek magical papyri, which are dated on the whole well down into the Roman period. His initial definition of magic is akin to the one we offer above (pp. 3–4). After enumerating the various invisible powers (including the gods, heroes, angels, demons, and the powers of such natural objects as plants, minerals, animals, with which the invisible powers are linked), he asserts: "The art of magic is to collect such knowledge and apply it correctly so as to swing the enormous forces of the universe in the desired direction."[26] But as his case unfolds, Hull broadens his definition of magic to include any sort of belief in angels and demons, while at the same time he plays down the importance of technique as the means by which the magician attends his ends.[27] The result is that any exorcism is automatically described as magical. The parallel evidence adduced by Hull is – inevitably – from the second and subsequent centuries; Lucian, Philostratus, the magical papyri. What Hull has ignored is that belief in angels and demons was operative in Judaism and in early Christianity in contexts where magic is not present or not a significant factor. Jewish apocalypticism assumes the existence and function of angels and demons. Yet the larger framework of meaning in which these superhuman beings are said to be at work is utterly different from the coercive, manipulative mood of the second and third centuries when magic was flourishing, as Peter Brown's brilliant analytical studies have shown.[28] To make historical judgments on the basis of arbitrary definitions or theological prejudices does not contribute to constructive inquiry. What Hull has ignored is that there is a fundamental difference between the apocalyptic worldview, which sees the cosmos as the place of struggle between God and his opponents, but which awaits the triumph of God and the vindication of his faithful people, and the magical view which regards the gods and all the other powers as fair game for exploitation and manipulation by those shrewd enough to achieve thereby their own ends or the defeat of their enemies. There is no hint of the latter outlook — which is the essence of magic — in the synoptic tradition or in its apocalyptic antecedents, but it becomes a pervasive factor of life in the Roman world from the Antonine period onward. It is precisely to this epoch that Hull must turn in his effort to document his position.

Although the later New Testament writings continue to value miracle as the evidence of God's action in human affairs, there begin to be traces of magic as well. In the Book of Acts, for example, there is evidence of the influence of magical technique, even though the basic outlook of the writer is religious, and most of the miracles fit the religious pattern. Magical features are apparent in some healing stories but especially in accounts of divine punitive action, which is a typical feature of magic. In the story of Ananias and Sapphira, for example, who withheld some of their possessions when all the members of the Christian community were pooling theirs, both are struck dead as a consequence of their disobedience (Acts 4:32–5:11).

The closest to the automatic or coercive magical forces that one finds in the gospel tradition is, perhaps, in the story of the woman with the bloody flow who touches Jesus as he passes and is healed (Lk 8:43–8), although Jesus is said there to be aware that power (δύναμις) had gone out of him. But in Acts 5:12–16, even the contact with the sick through Peter's shadow falling on them effects healing. Akin to this is the account in Acts 19:11 that healings and exorcisms were accomplished through handkerchiefs and aprons which Peter had touched and which then were efficacious healing instruments. This is a prime example of what John Ferguson, in his study, *The Religions of the Roman Empire*,[29] has called the magical power of "the extended personality", by which possession of or contact with a part of a person, even his name, is the medium of sharing in his power or in exercising power over him. In Acts 28:1–10, the story of Paul's being bitten by a viper shows that the people of Malta were expecting a punitive miracle, but instead God vindicates Paul by enabling him to go unharmed from the attack. The effort of Herod Agrippa (Acts 12:20–3) to have himself acclaimed as divine results in his being struck down by a gruesome fatal disease — an account which is roughly paralleled in Josephus' description of his death (*Antiquities* xix.8.2). Although these stories border on magic, Luke seems to be telling them to demonstrate that God is in control of history and of human life, rather than as a self-contained demonstration of magical technique. In Acts 8, however, Simon — whose special designation is Magus! — first abandoned his own lucrative trade as a magician because of the superior power of the Holy Spirit. When he tried to purchase the gift of the Spirit, however, he was severely rebuked (Acts 8:9–24). What is significant is that in Acts there is clear evidence that the power of the Holy Spirit and that of magic are seen to be in competition, beginning with the launching of the mission of the church to the Gentiles. The charges that are brought against Paul and his associates centre on magical practices, as shown by the story of the opposition from a Jewish magician (Acts 13:6–12), the accusation brought when Paul expels a "spirit of divination" from a slave girl in Ephesus (Acts 16:16–18), and the burning of the magic books when their former users are converted (Acts 19:13–19).

We have already noted how keen the competition was between Peter and Simon Magus in the second-century document, The Acts of Peter. In the Clementine Recognitions (II.5–16) Simon is denounced as a false, self-promoting teacher and practiser of magic. He claims to be able to perform signs and prodigies, to pass through rocks and fire, and to transform persons and animals into other forms. Although he claims to do these exploits by the power of God, in fact he is in league with the spirits of the dead. The Christians are at pains to discredit Simon, who is portrayed as the archetype of those who perform what they allege to be miracles, often in competition with the claims of the Christian miracle workers. As E.R. Dodds has observed, the controversy over miracle and magic in the Roman world of the second and third centuries was not a debate between believers and rationalists, but between two different sorts of believers. Fear of magic was not confined to the ignorant. Men as highly educated as Plotinus and Libanius seriously believed themselves to have been the objects of magical attack. It is not surprising, therefore, that the early Christian apologists "had little to say about the personality of Jesus or about the doctrine of the atonement. Instead, they placed their main reliance on two arguments which their present-day successors have in general abandoned – the argument from miracles and the argument from prophecy."[30]

It is through Origen's *Contra Celsum* that we have our best access to the seriousness and the substance of the intellectual debate between Christians and those seeking earnestly to preserve the heritage of the pagan tradition – especially in its Greek mode – in the face of mounting threat from Christianity. In Celsus' polemic against Christianity, and especially against the representation of Jesus in the gospel tradition, we see how the lines were drawn. Origen's excerpts from Celsus' ἀληθὴς λόγος are sufficiently full that the basic argument and detailed strategy of the latter's work are clear in Origen's apologetic response.[31] Following the classic analysis of this debate by Carl Andresen, in *Logos und Nomos: Die Polemick Kelsos wider das Urchristentum*,[32] three recent studies analyse the differences in philosophical, social and cultural outlook which underlie this debate and which work to generate the specifics of the argument: Harold Remus, *Pagan–Christian Conflict over Miracle in the Second Century*;[33] Eugene V. Gallagher, *Divine Man or Magician? Celsus and Origen on Jesus*;[34] Robert L. Wilken, *The Christians as the Romans Saw Them*.[35]

All of these studies recognize that the point at issue between Celsus and the Christians was not a matter of doctrine or merely of theological preference, but involved different basic stances adopted toward traditional Graeco-Roman culture. As Wilken phrases it, drawing on Andresen, Christianity was beginning to create a counterculture which threatened the cohesion and stability of society, and which worked for the dissolution of the norms of law and rationality on which Celsus' own Middle Platonic culture was based, consciously and unconsciously.[36] The antipathy toward Christianity evident in Celsus' attack is grounded on his perception that in abandoning traditional social and intellectual principles, Christianity had the potential for undermining the ways of thinking and acting which were foundational to Roman society in the second century. He does not deny the possibility that the extraordinary may and does occur, but he rejects flatly the Christian explanation of those miraculous events. His attack on the Christians is often expressed through a Jewish polemicist, although elsewhere Celsus betrays his own hostility toward Judaism as well. Precisely because the Christians in the second century are building their case for their faith on the claims of miracles being performed and prophecy being fulfilled through Jesus, it is on these issues that Celsus concentrates his attack. Celsus, in spite of his appeal to *logos*, does not come across to the reader as a rationalist who makes no place for the supernatural, but writes as one whose cultural values and assumptions are fundamentally incompatible with those of the Christians.

Celsus begins his attack — or at least Origen begins his excerpting of Celsus' polemic — by scorning the social status of the movement and of its founder. Since by Roman law all secret societies are illegal, the secret movement that is Christianity exists contrary to Roman law (*Contra Celsum* I.1). The founder of the movement, Jesus, was the illegitimate son of a poor country woman, who, "after she has been driven out by her husband and while she was wandering about in a disgraceful way ... secretly gave birth to Jesus". He did not rise above his miserable origins, but, "because he was poor, hired himself out as a workman in Egypt, and there he tried his hand at certain magical powers on which the Egyptians pride themselves; he returned [to Palestine] full of conceit because of these powers, and on account of them gave himself the title of God" (I.29). Not surprisingly, the intelligent were put off by his teachings (III.73), and he attracted to himself followers who were uneducated (III.44), the young and ignorant (III.50, 55), those who were violators of civil and moral laws (III.59), and the boorish and the seditious (VIII.49). If any credence were to have been given to his claims, his post-resurrection appearances ought to have taken place in the presence of credible witnesses (II.63, 67) instead of a group of hysterical women (II.55).

Like the Jews in the books of the Bible, on which the Christians based their claims about Jesus, the leaders of the Christian movement must be traced back to sorcerers. Apparently Celsus is making his analogy here on the basis of the magical papyri, which include the names of Jesus as well as Adonai, Iao, and other divine designations taken from the biblical tradition. Celsus does not call into question the Christian claim that by Jesus and through his name extraordinary feats were performed. For him the crucial factor is to attribute these to magic, rather than to the more traditional factor of miracle associated particularly with Asklepios, whom Celsus obviously holds in high regard (III.22–3). He is certain that there were, in the Greek tradition, certain human beings who were raised to the rank of the immortals, and whose acts of beneficence and mystical appearances continue to be experienced down to his own time. He contrasts this with Jesus, who appears only to his own circle of followers and whose benefactions are limited to the faithful. He is quite prepared to believe the claims of "a great multitude of men, both of Greeks and barbarians, [who] confess that they have often seen and still do see not just a phantom, but Asklepios himself healing men and doing good and predicting the future" (III.24). Celsus is willing to believe in miracles, but not to attribute them to Jesus, who is low class and attracts low class followers. Origen's response is to point out the benefits that flow to humanity through Jesus and to assert the prophecies which have been fulfilled about Jesus and by Jesus. For Celsus, however, Asklepios is a true manifestation of the divine in human form, while Jesus is an imposter (VII.35).

The miracles which the Christians attribute to Jesus have as their model, Celsus declares, the stunts of Egyptian sorcerers. Celsus compares the story of Jesus' feeding the five thousand with "the accomplishments of those who are taught by the Egyptians, who for a few obols make known their sacred lore in the middle of the marketplace and drive daemons out of men and blow away diseases and invoke the souls of heroes, displaying expensive banquets and dining-tables and cakes and dishes which are non-existent, and who make things move as though they were alive although they are not really so, but only appear as such in the imagination". Origen notes with accuracy that Celsus does indeed believe in magic, but he goes on to make the distinction between a magician who puts on public stunts like these in order to gain money and a following, and Jesus, whose miracles are performed for the benefit of the human race and as the basis for instruction of his followers in the ways of God (I.68). Celsus argues elsewhere (II.49–51) that since Jesus acknowledged that others were doing works similar to his own, his charge that they performed their miracles as sorcerers and by the powers of evil must be applied equally to his own marvellous acts. To this Origen responds that extraordinary deeds can originate from divine or from diabolical powers: it is up to the careful observer to recognize the source of the power. Just as Moses' people saw in him the agent of God for their deliverance and preservation, so the Christians have the discernment to recognize in Jesus God's instrument for their salvation.

The specifics of Celsus's belief in sorcery are evident in his charge that the Christians are able to perform their extraordinary deeds "by pronouncing the names of certain demons and incantations" (I.6). Or again, in VI.39, he declares that the Christians "use some sort of magic and sorcery and invoke certain demons with barbarous names ... while invoking the same demons in various languages [they] bamboozle people who do not know that their names have one form among the Greeks and another form among the Scythians". The reference here may be to the magical formulae (known to us from the magical papyri) or to the formulations of the Gnostics. But in either case, these invocations of strange names were not part of standard Christian practice. And in any event, they show Celsus as anything but sceptical about the reality and the potency of magical practices.

The crux of Celsus' attack on Christianity and its claims concerning the miracles of Jesus appears when he gives his estimate of who Jesus is and what his acts signify. How is one to evaluate the figure of Jesus? For Celsus he was not the great prince and lord of the earth expected by the Jewish prophets (II.28–9), but a "pestilential fellow" who brought no benefits to humanity and no light of knowledge of the divine (II.30). Instead of the Logos pure and holy whom Christians claim Jesus to be, he is only "a man who was arrested most disgracefully and crucified" (II.31). Origen responds by calling attention not only to the fact that "to this day people whom God wills are cured by his name", but also to a factor of great significance for Romans of this period, as attested by the frequency of its occurrence in the historians of the early centuries of our era: portents. The eclipse, the darkness, the tearing of the temple veil, and the earthquakes are all reported in the gospels (especially Matthew) as indicators of the change of power on the earth.[37] In the Roman sources these portents point to the birth or impending death of a ruler or a dynasty. Origen makes a comparable claim for them, as is implied in Matthew's gospel, about the birth and death of Jesus and the portents that accompanied those events. The debate is not over whether the gods give portents; the issue is what these reported events in the Jesus tradition portend.

Celsus betrays at certain points his own ambivalence about the claims which the Christians make for Jesus, just as he has high words of praise for the wisdom of civilizations other than the Greek (Chaldean, Egyptian, Persian, even with reservations, the Jews; VI.80). One gets the impression that, even if Celsus were to have to admit that Jesus and the Christians were not fakes but actually performed extraordinary acts, he wants it to be clear that all such earthly activities are eclipsed in importance by the eternal realities to which he as a (Middle) Platonist is primarily committed (VIII.60):

> We must, however, be careful about this, lest by association with these beings anyone should become absorbed in the healing with which they are concerned, and by becoming a lover of the body and turning away from higher things should be held down without realizing it. For perhaps we ought not to disbelieve wise men who say that most of the earthly demons are absorbed with created things, and are riveted to blood and burnt-offering and magical enchantments, and are bound to this sort of thing, and can do nothing better than healing the body and predicting the coming fortune of men and cities, and that all their knowledge and power concerns merely mortal activities.

As Harold Remus has shown, Celsus' argument is not neatly consistent. The parallels between what he says about Asklepios and what the Christians claim for Jesus are evident: both were notable healers, both were powerless in the face of death; both were sub-sequently exalted; both became the central figures in cults through which healings were performed. Celsus plays down the theme of the resurrection of Asklepios, since it does not fit in with his basically Platonic point of view, and this enables him to scoff at the resurrection of Jesus. But he cannot reject miracle on principle; he can only dismiss those attributed to Jesus by denouncing them as frauds. At issue between Celsus and the Christians is the choice between two symbolic universes: the one transmitted from Greek classical culture through the Hellenistic and Roman periods, and embodied in the view of the world adopted in the period of the Second Sophistic. The stress falls on the continuity of traditional wisdom, the process of transmission of knowledge through the established Greek patterns of instruction and learning, the preservation of the values of the intellectual élite, and especially of the Platonic valuing of the realm of the eternal. Celsus sees this life-world as not only incompatible with the emerging Christian views of society, history and cosmology, but as profoundly threatened by this new competitor. Even though he shares with the Christians the belief that the transcendent discloses itself in visible, tangible form in the phenomenal world, he abhors the bourgeois cast of characters that dominate the Christian story, the lack of intellectual sophistication which characterizes their way of thinking, and the non-Greek origin of their outlook on life and their hopes for the future. Accordingly, he is driven to discredit the entire enterprise, including its origins, its claims, and its aspirations. At stake for him is the preservation of what he regarded as authentic culture and society, stemming out of Greek tradition.

5

CONCLUDING OBSERVATIONS

E. R. Dodds' observation, quoted above, on the importance for early
Christian apologists of miracle and prophecy, is both accurate and
important for the historical analysis of this period.[1] It has a direct
bearing on the relationships among the three sets of phenomena with
which we are concerned in this study: medicine, miracle, and magic.
All three are modes of achieving or sustaining human welfare. All
manifest methods for dealing with the universal problems of human
suffering and death, and by extension with the problem of evil. Each
assumes the existence and operation of some system of order which
can be perceived, understood and exploited in order to attain a
maximum of benefit for those who have the wisdom to utilize these
resources. Yet the assumptions on which each system operates are
significantly different.

Medicine builds on the foundation of natural order. The goal
of the physician is to discern the patterns of the natural functioning
of the human body, by direct observation where possible, by analogy
from the organisms which can be studied at first hand, and by
inference from the philosophical principles of cosmic order which
experience and reason have led him to adopt as normative. The
study of the environment – topography, weather, flora, fauna
– provides the physician with the means for aiding the healthy
function of the human organism or for avoiding those factors
which are injurious to health. This includes change of climate or
place of residence, and use of natural substances to assist or correct
the bodily functions. There are certain acknowledged limits to the
effectiveness of this procedure, such as certain diseases which are
admitted to be beyond the power of surgery or therapy to overcome.
And there is the – mostly tacit – recognition of the temporal
limits of human life. But within those limits, medicine seeks to
increase the effectiveness of its service to human health and the
extension and happiness of human life. Beyond these wide horizons

there is the, also usually tacit, acknowledgment that human destiny is in the hands of the gods.

Those who claim to see or to experience miracle assume a different system of cosmic order. For them, the gods – or God – are in control, working out a divine purpose in the creation for the benefit of all the creatures. To the faithful seekers, the gods disclose that purpose through divination and prophecy. To those who come seeking help or remedy in situations of special need, the gods respond directly, with the result that there occurs recovery of the lost, or regaining of health, or restoration of limbs, or sight, or hearing. These acts of divine beneficence may be perceived as purely personal, containing their ends within the events themselves, or they may be seen as pointing to the fulfilment of the encompassing divine scheme, as is the case with the exorcisms in early Christian tradition which point to the defeat of the powers of evil and the establishment of God's Rule in the world. For others, the larger meaning of miracle may have to do not merely with the momentary recovery of health, but with the awareness of and progress toward the goal of one's life, as in the case of Aristides' exaltation as rhetorician. In distinction from the medical point of view, with its primary interest in the discovery and maintenance of natural order, the worldview implicit in miracle conceives of the divine as personal, and therefore seeks to conform life to the will of the god(s). Since there are persons and forces at work in the world which seek to thwart the divine plan, the god(s) must on occasion intervene in punitive fashion, in order to bring to an end those persons or those activities which stand in the way of the cosmic purpose. The believer in miracle seeks to attune life and to sharpen perception in harmony with the divine will.

In the realm of magic the basic assumption is that there is a mysterious, inexorable network of forces which the initiated can exploit for personal benefit, or block for personal protection. These forces have acquired many names. The well-informed will utilize the power inherent in those names in order to achieve desired ends. Like the operator at the controls of a powerful modern machine, the forces are resident in the cosmos. The questions are: Who will use them? For what ends? The magician has at his disposal a kind of operator's manual, by means of which he can bend the forces to serve his own will, whether for his own benefit or for the defeat of his opponents. There is not in view any overall picture or set of goals, neither the inherent natural order of a Stoic-dominated culture, nor the escha-tologically oriented assumptions of the biblical tradition, nor the mystical image of a life in association with the gods. There is no need to understand the specifics of the powers themselves. Rather, the viewpoint is pragmatic: What is it that will make the system work for the purposes of the operator?

As we have seen, in practice the lines are not always so sharply drawn. Adjacent to the medical schools of Cos and Pergamum are the shrines where incubation occurs and direct healings take place. The miracle workers engage in practices which border on magic in their impersonal efficacy. The magical formulae invoke the names of the miracle-working deities. Even Galen will permit the use of magical amulets when medical technique fails.[2] Indeed the Hippocratic tradition describes medical discoveries as made by those who "pursuing their inquiries excellently and with suitable application of reason to the nature of man, made their discoveries, and thought their art worthy to be ascribed to a god, as in fact is the usual belief" (Hippocrates I.37). Yet even when it is inferred that ancient physicians believed that their medical insights were the gift of the gods,[3] it is clear that a different view of the gods is operative from that inherent in the belief in miracle. If the focus is on inherent natural order as the means to retaining or regaining health, we are in the realm of medicine. If it is on the divine will at work in human experience, concerned for human destiny and cosmic purpose, then we are in the realm of miracle. If it is on an impersonal system which will operate in response to the one skilled in the use of coercive power, then we are in the realm of magic. Superficial similarities with regard to details in each of these realms must not lead us to confusion or to blurring distinctions. Responsibility to historical evidence requires that we differentiate the basic outlook which lies behind, inheres in, and informs the claims that are made with regard to these three different modes of attaining human well-being.

What is the bearing of these historical observations concerning medicine, miracle and magic on interpreting the New Testament? The first conclusion is that the phenomenon of healing in the gospels and elsewhere in the New Testament is a central factor in primitive Christianity, and was so from the beginning of the movement. It is not a later addendum to the tradition, introduced in order to make Jesus more appealing to the Hellenistic world, but was a major feature of the Jesus tradition from the outset. Indeed, it is almost certainly a part of the historical core of that tradition, even though it is likely to have been embellished in the process of transmission. The performance of miracles in first-century Judaism is adequately attested even though the significance given to it in the Jesus tradition – signs of the inbreaking of the New Age – is a distinctive development of the apocalyptic tradition of Judaism, especially as we see it in Daniel. As the gospels attest, and as the evidence of the Hellenistic healing cults suggests, the performance of healings and exorcisms by Jesus was seen as a central factor in the rapidly developed movement that Jesus called forth in Palestine and Syria, as well as in the astonishing spread of Christianity throughout the Mediterranean world.

This leads to a second observation: the role of Jesus as healer was by no means an accommodation of an itinerant preacher–prophet to Hellenistic culture, but was in direct continuity with the Old Testament prophetic understanding of what God was going to do in the New Age, for the salvation of his people and for the healing of the nations. Jesus is pictured in the gospel tradition as pre-eminently the agent of Yahweh the Healer – a theological perspective which reaches back to the Exodus and pervades the prophetic tradition, as we have noted above. The evidence of the post-exilic concern for healing is apparent in such so-called inter-testamental writings as Sirach, and in the Dead Sea Scrolls (4Q Therapeia). The ability to perform wonders, including healings, figures importantly in Paul's apologia for his apostolic ministry.

The ostensibly negative factor that miracle as eschatological sign does not figure in the later rabbinic tradition of miracle-working is important: it suggests that in the parting of the ways which took place in the late first century between the two developing movements – rabbinic Judaism and early Christianity – it was the former group which looked to miracle as confirmation of authority in the interpretation of the law, while the Christians saw in miracles evidence of the coming of God's Rule. As in the case of the emergence of their respective canons of scripture, and in their differing interpretations of the law (as evident especially in Matthew's heightening of the difference in the Sermon on the Mount)[4] there seems to have been a kind of agreement to disagree on the meaning of miracle. But the differences in significance of this phenomenon heighten the importance of the factor itself, rather than moving it to the periphery as certain scholars have sought to do. Although the primary importance of miracle in the New Testament is that of eschatological sign, it is also interpreted symbolically, especially in the Gospel of John, along lines broadly analogous to Plutarch's handling of the Isis mythology, as we have observed. This approach to miracle frees the interpreter from literalistic acceptance of the miracle stories at face value – an approach which Plutarch explicitly rejects in favour of his symbolic hermeneutical process. The early Christians who were so inclined obviously felt free to adopt the same interpretive method. Miracle becomes in John the symbol of spiritual renewal, of mystical participation, of sustenance, of insight. The healing works of Jesus are means to spiritual transformation rather than ends in themselves.

The portrayal of healing in the New Testament stands on the whole in sharp contrast to magic. In our survey of medicine, however, we noted how overt commitment to purely medical modes of therapy or to the type of natural remedy called for by Pliny in practice shades over into magic at times. Similarly, in the apocryphal gospels and Acts, the miracle stories told about Jesus and the apostle take on the features of magical practice, for both healing and punitive ends. Within the New Testament writings we can see the beginning of this kind of development. It accelerates rapidly in some of the later Christian writings and especially in the Gnostic traditions, as the Gnostic writings and the magical papyri abundantly attest. There is in the gospel narratives no trace of the elaborate multi-named invocations of the gods, the agglomerations of nonsense letters and syllables, the coercive manipulations of the unseen powers which characterize the magical papyri. The aim of the healing is not to force the gods to act but to share in the fulfilment of God's purpose in the creation and for his people.

What remains central in the New Testament, in spite of real differences in perspective among the writers and the communities that they address, is the conviction that God is alone in control of human destiny, even though the powers of Satan have for a time seized control or sought to thwart the divine plan. That plan is being accomplished through an agent whom God has chosen and empowered. The analogies between the miracle tradition in the New Testament and that found in the Exodus narratives is obvious: the signs which God has sent to effect the liberation of his people (Ex 10:1–2) have been performed through Aaron (Ex 8:6). Yahweh calls his covenant people to obedience in his capacity as "Yahweh your healer" (Ex 15:26). In the New Testament counterpart to these signs, addressed to the people of the New Covenant, there is likewise an assurance that the plan of Yahweh the Healer is being achieved through the signs that God's agents perform. The first and paradigmatic agent is Jesus; then, by the power he bestows, his followers as well. A fundamental difference from the perspective on miracle as eschatological sign in post-exilic Judaism, including both Daniel and the Qumran documents, is that the invitation to share in God's healing actions is not limited to those who have preserved ritual purity. Rather, the bounds of participation in the benefits of Yahweh the healer are open to all who, though Jesus, turn to God in trust. The divine redemptive purpose and the instrument of its accomplishment are, therefore, best epitomized in the Q saying of Jesus, "If, indeed, it is by the finger of God that I cast out demons, then the kingdom of God has come upon you" (Lk 11:20).

APPENDIX

James H. Charlesworth
George L. Collord Professor of New Testament
Princeton Theological Seminary

4Q Therapeia (43.407)
Cryptic Notes on the Medical Rounds of Omriel

A New Text and Translation

* * * * *

In a sensational – indeed polemical – book, J. M. Allegro has printed "a hitherto unpublished document from the Fourth Cave cache, 4 Q Therapeia" (p. 7). I have decided to offer a new reading of the text with a translation because it is apparent that its existence is virtually unknown, even to scholars, and because few of them would be perusing such a book as Allegro's *The Dead Sea Scrolls and the Christian Myth* (Newton Abbot: Westbridge Books, 1979; repr., New York: Prometheus Books, 1984). Furthermore, the discernment of the consonants and the resulting translation can be improved over Allegro's initial publication.

Allegro's transcription and translation[1] are as follows:

Transcription

1 lk'ps 'ṣgdḥw [...] šẏk̇l
2 sḥrh 'l̇ẏṩ' 'k̇sṅẇs ṫṙṡẏ
3 tyrqẇs [...]' by' .[...]q
4 šdḥsw mgns mlkyh mnws
5 mḥtyš mqlyḥ mpybšt
6 ḃġlgws bnwbn bsry gdy
7 dlwy hlkws hrqnws yny w
8 ytr'ytyšyl' zwḥlwlp
8ᵃ yṫrws ysy
9 'qwl' zkry'l yṅy
10 'ly 'dpy
10ᵃ 'mry'l qp[...]

Translation

1 The report of the Caiaphas (*Qayy'phā'*), being an account of
2 his rounds of the afflicted (among) the guests: supplies of
3 medicines [...] [...] swelling [...]
4 which distended him through a kind of flabbiness due to wasting: –

5   a braying of stalks of 'Mephibosheth'
6   in the smegma (found) in the sheaths of the penes of kids.
7   The ulcer of Hyrcanus Yannai was drawn and
8   the secretions pertaining to it that were discharging; also for
8ᵃ Peter Yosai;
9   Colic – Zachariel Yannai;
10 Eli is witness, dictated by
10ᵃ Omriel, QP (*Qayy'phā'*?)

Methodology

The first task is to date the script of this fragment. The writing is clearly Herodian, with features from formal and late Herodian. This script is strikingly similar to 4QDanᵇ (*c* A.D. 20–50) and to 4QDeutʲ (*c* A.D. 50).[2] Its date, therefore, is probably sometime between A.D. 30 and 50. By studying Cross's typology of these scripts it is possible to discern potentially ambiguous consonants; only through paleographical analysis (of the whole text and of separate forms) can I distinguish, *inter alia*, a *Hē* from a *Ḥēth*, *Dāleth* from *Rēsh*, *Yōdh* from *Wāw*, and *Bēth* from *Kaph*.

Second, it is essential to observe the quality and state of preservation of the leather on which the document was written. It is virtually indecipherable, except through infrared photography (compare the photographs in Allegro, *Myth*, p. 128; the 1979 edition is clearer; the best photograph is in my *4Q Therapeia*, see note 5 below). The leather is also creased, so that some of the consonants are difficult to discern. As a result, the following reconstruction needs to be improved by a study of the document itself. (A visit to Jerusalem failed to locate the document; it seems to be misplaced.)

Third, the move from mute forms to discernible meaning must be guided by a judgment about the purpose and intent of the fragment. Focusing initially only on the words that are clear and possess unambiguous meanings helps in this process. The words that require no speculative guesswork or emendation are the following:[3]

Line	1 *lk'ps*	for (or by) Caiaphas
	2 *shrh*	his itinerary
	3 *tyřqí ' bwⁱ*	medicines (A) an abscess
	4 *šdḥsw mqns mlkyh mnws*	his pressure from a kind of nausea from sickness (?)
	5 *mḥtwš tqlyh mpybšt*	... offence of Mephibosheth
	6 .... *gdy*	a kid
	7 .... *hlkws hrqnws yny w*	... the wound of Hyrcanus Yannai and
	8 *ytr 'ytẘšyl' zwḥlwlp*	the secretions belonging to it, the ones flowing, and for P
	9 *ytṛws ysy*	etros Yose[4]
	10 *'qwl' zkry'l yṅy*	Aquila, Zachariel Yannai
	11 *'ly 'rpw*	Eli, the back of his neck
(*ex margine*) *°mṙy'l qp*	Omriel *qp* (?)

From this preliminary examination two aspects of the writing should guide our decipherment. The cryptic note reports the medical rounds of a physician named Omriel. The abundant feature of nouns ending in *ws* reveals that we will be dealing with loan words, almost always from the Greek language, and that interpretation – from reading consonants to exegesis – must be informed by insights derived from a non-Semitic, especially Greek, culture.

One of the keys to decipherment is reading out loud a group of consonants. Often the author confuses similar sounding consonants, such as *Gimel* and *Zayin* (how could he confuse these two distinct Semitic sounds, or was he poorly trained in writing?) in line one; *Ḥēth* for *Kaph* in line 5; *Nūn* for *Zayin* in line 6 (did he have a problem in hearing or pronouncing a *Nūn*?); and *Sāmekh* for *Sîn* in line 6. Also by hearing the writings read aloud one can recall words in other languages, such as Greek, Syriac, Arabic, and Latin. Only by appealing to these languages is interpretation of this document possible; after all, it is characterized by transliterations. By employing the methodology just summarized in the preceding paragraphs, I have been able to reconstruct and interpret this cryptic note. Here are the transcription and translation:

Transcription

```
 1  lkʿps ʾs̆g̊dhw šk̊wl
 2  shrh ʾlyṣ̊ ʾksn̊ws̆ t̊[r]s̊[y]
 3  tyr̊qt̊ ʾ bwⁱ q
 4  šdḥsw mgns mlkyh mnws
 5  mḥtwš tglyh mpybšt
 6  b̊g̊lgws bnwbn bsry gdy
 7  dlwy hlkws hrqnws yny w
 8  ytrʾytẘšylʾ zwḥlwlp
 9  yṭrws ysy
10  ʿqwlʾ zkryʾl yn̊y
11  ʿly ʿrpw
(ex margine) ⁱmr̊yʾl qp̊
```

Translation

 1 For Caiaphas, (from) his messenger (Omriel) concerning all of
 2 his itinerary. The afflicted (among) the strangers he supplied
 3 (with) medicines. An abscess (was found in one of the strangers). q.
 4 The pressure (on) his (abdomen resulted) from a kind of nausea (from) sickness.
 5 (Another stranger suffered) from crushed (limbs like) the offense of Mephibosheth
 6 With the milky liquid from the testicles in the scrotum of a kid
 7 he (i.e., Omriel) drew (out of the water and cleansed) the wound of Hyrcanus Yannai; and
 8 the secretions belonging to it (especially the) ones (actively) flowing. And (he applied the same remedy) for P-
 9 etros Yose,
10 Aquila, (and) Zachariel Yannai;

11 (also the same treatment was given to) Eli (except the wound was on the) back of his neck.

(*ex margine*) (By) Omriel: (Report number) 180.

Significance of the Fragment

This appendix serves merely to introduce the fragment and represents an attempt to interpret it. This is not the place for a full consideration of the importance of the fragment, but it should be noted that we have in this document a medical testimony that not merely derives, but also dates from the period between Hippocrates and Galen. The influence from the Greek world is striking, and raises the question: How much and what kind of medical knowledge was available in Judea and Galilee before A.D. 70?

It is my impression that the patients − all of them men − had suffered in some 'battle'. Why were these individuals wounded? Why was this document placed in Cave 4? In the future I shall suggest a possible scenario behind these lines.[5]

Line 1. *lk'ps*; Allegro thinks the *l* is a *lamedh auctoris*: "The report of the Caiaphas (*Qayy^ephā'*)." This interpretation is possible, but I think the report is from Omriel to Caiaphas. The former name is in the margin; there is no reason to equate the two names; "his messenger" in line 1 indicates someone other than Caiaphas; and the note is in the third person, whereas one would have expected notes to oneself to be in the first person. The *Kaph* in this name actually looks like a *Bēth*; our author's writing is inelegant and unrefined.

'ṣġdhw. This reading is an error for *'yzgdhw*. See *'îzgadh*, "a runner, messenger." Allegro correctly points to Persian *iskudār*, "postman"; but he prefers "his message, report". That reading demands another form of the word: cf. Syriac, *'îgadûthâ*, "message."

škwl; partly worn away. Perhaps the rabbinic *Shîn* with "all".

Line 2. *'lyṣ'*; a guess; cf. Syriac, *'âlîṣâ*, "afflicted, oppressed".

'ksṅwś. A conjecture based on days of reading this fragment without interruption. Cf. Greek *xenos* and Syriac *'āks^enāi*, "stranger, guest, foreigner".

t̊[r]š[y]; cf. Syriac, *tarsî*, "he nourished, supplied". See Odes of Solomon 16:2.

Line 3. *tyṙgí* or *tyṙgwś*; this form is difficult and it is impossible to be certain given the state of the manuscript and photograph. The initial *Tāw* is clear. It is followed by a *Wāw* or a *Yōdh*. These are written similarly in this text. The *Rēsh* seems likely. The *Qōph* is certain.

The final *Tāw* or *Wāw* and *Sāmekh* are problematic. The *Wāw* may have been written poorly or have been altered by the creased leather. The *Sāmekh* may be partly worn away. It can be argued that it is separate from a preceding *Wāw*, or that a crease in the leather (or subsequent falling away of the ink) causes the *Tāw* to look separated.

The *Wāw* can begin another word (see lines 8 and 9 in which a new word begins without being separated and is then incorrectly divided and separated from one line to the next). See the suggestion below.

There are three possibilities: (1) *tyrgws* conceivably represents the Greek *thēriakos*, which evolved, perhaps by the first century, from meaning "concerning venomous beasts" to "antidotes" and to "drugs".

(2) *tyrg* would transliterate the Greek feminine noun *thēriakē*, "antidote, medicine". This Greek noun is transliterated into rabbinic Hebrew (*tyryyg'* [Sabbath 109b]) and Syriac (*teryagê*). I would expect the final Greek *ē* to be represented; but in some Galilean inscriptions it is ignored. See *prwṭwn*, which represents Greek *prōtōnē*, and *glnyq*, which transliterates the Greek *kallinikē* respectively in ggHA 1.3 and ggHA 3.1. Note that Syriac *tôryāgâ* is a transliteration of Greek *tēriakon*, "medicine". This same process could produce *twrg* in line 3. I prefer *tyrg*.

A following *ws* may begin another word and be linked with a *Lāmedh*, the top of which is perhaps still visible on the bottom of line 2. This could represent the remains of a *wšl[q']*, which could be *w^esalqā'*, perhaps a transliteration of Greek *salka*, "a fragrant oil". This speculative reconstruction would produce the following: "The afflicted (among) the strangers he supplied (with) medicine and oi[l]."

(3) *tyṙqî* may represent the Greek feminine noun *thēriakē* – as above – with a Semitic feminine ending *Tāw*, which could be a construct (unlikely) or plural: "medicines". There is certainly no reason to demand or expect a full writing (*tyrqwt*) for this form. This third possibility is most likely; it is the simplest solution and allows for the idiosyncratic, rapid and unpolished manner of writing.

This text is a difficult one. It demands imagination and some speculation. I look forward to learning from others, and improving these suggestions and speculations.

bw^i; Allegro: *by'*; but that form means "rejoicing". *bw'* denotes "swelling, abscess."

Line 4. *šdḥsw*; literally, "his pressure" (i.e., on the abdomen; cf. Yebamoth 42a). The pressure is probably not caused by a physician feeling for a cure; it is rather some pressure caused by an illness in or injury to the patient.

mgns; from Greek, *genos*, "order, kind, sort".

mlkyh; usually *malakhyâ*, from Greek *malakia*, "want of appetite, nausea".

mnws; according to Allegro, "from wasting", but his reading of line 4 is unconvincing. This form is not *mānôs*, "flight, escape, refuge". It is probably not a faulty transliteration from the Greek, *nosos*, "disease". The author would have added the ending here, as elsewhere. It is probably from Aramaic *n^esas*, "to be sick"; cf. Aramaic *nûš*, Assyrian *nasâsu*, "to wail, lament", and Syriac *nas*, "to be weak, infirm, sickly". Contrast, however, Arabic, *nws*, "to move to and fro", and Syriac, *nas*,[2] "to tremble".

Line 5. Allegro: "a braying of stalks of Mephibosheth." I find this translation opaque.

mḥtwš; an error for *mktwš*, probably a passive participle from *kathaš*, "to crush". Mephibosheth was lame in both feet (cf. 2 Samuel 9:13); the patient in this text had two crushed limbs (or ankles), so that like Mephibosheth he was doubly lame. The patient could have suffered from an injury while involved in heavy labour, such as moving the heavy stones to the Temple. If these strangers are soldiers (see lines 6–11), then he may have been run over by a chariot or clubbed.

tqlyh; see *taqlayyâ*, "an offense, stumbling block". Mephibosheth, the son of Jonathan, was cursed by being lame in both feet. He had been dropped by his nurse (2 Samuel 4:4). This lameness could be regarded as the result of someone's offence or transgression (Saul's?), or perhaps it is described as offensive to behold. The initial *Tāw* is marred by the crease.

Line 6. *bg̊lgws*; a transliteration of Greek, *glagos*, "milk".

bnwbn; an error for *bzwbn*: *zūbbān* is the bag which contains a male animal's sexual organs; the scrotum. Contrast Allegro, "the sheaths of the penes". His interpretation overlooks the medicinal quality of the testicle's liquid: it would be sterile. The opposite would be true of Allegro's rendering of the text. Also, there is an enzyme which possesses medical qualities in the testes' liquid; see my "Speculations on the Medical Sophistication of Omriel" in *The Discovery* (see note 5).

bsry; an error for *bśry*; *bśr* is the flesh, and can be a euphemism for penis (so Allegro). Here it is in the plural construct form. Kids have one penis but two testicles.

Line 7. *dlwy*; this form could be *dlww*, in which case see Latin *diluo*, "to wash apart, dissolve". But the form is probably related to *dālāh*, which in Hebrew, Aramaic and Syriac denotes, "to draw (water)", "to draw (out, with *min*)": cf. Assyrian *dalû*, *dilûtu*, "bucket", as well as English, "dilute". The action described seems to be the sponging or wiping clean of a wound; that is, to draw out the infected moisture and to cleanse the wound. The author is hampered not so much by the weakness of his own vocabulary as by the paucity of technical medical language in the language of his time.

hlkws; a transliteration of Greek *helkos*, "wound, ulcer".

yny; the *Nūn* was not written in its final form and then corrected; the Lāmedh from line 8 intrudes into the space for the *Nūn*.

w; the author incorrectly separates the *Wāw* from its noun. Was he influenced by the Greek *kai*?

Line 8. *ytr'ytŵśyl'* should have been *wytr'wtŵ*, "and its secretions"; see Syriac *yatîrᵉwāthâ*, "secretions, products", and *śyl'* or *śylh* (but *'Āleph* and *Hē* interchange in the Qumran Scrolls), "which to it".

zwḥlwlp should be divided: *zwḥl*; *wlp* goes with the next line. The *Wāw* before "Petros" looks like, but is not, a *Zayin*.

Line 9. *yṭrws*; restoring the separated consonants: *wlpyṭrws*, which renders the Greek, *Petros*.

Line 10. In contrast to Allegro, who misnumbers the lines of the fragment, I take these to represent proper names.

Line 11. *'rpw*, from *'ōreph*, "back of the neck". Contrast Allegro, "Eli is witness", based on his reading *'dpy*. The *Rēsh* and *Wāw* seem clear.

Ex margine: *qp*, which is not an abbreviated *Qayyᵉphā'*; Allegro claims that this name was written in the margin and abbreviated because of the "shortage of usable skin". But the photograph reveals ample space; and in line 1 Caiaphas is written with a *k* not a *q*. The form *qp* could mean a number; that is, the 180th report by Omriel. It is possible that *qn*, rather than *qr* was written, which would give the number 150.

NOTES

A list of translations of the primary sources will be found in the bibliography

Introduction

1 For example, *Gospel Parallels*, ed. B.H. Throckmorton. New York: Nelson, [1949], 1957.
2 See H.C. Kee, *Miracle in the Early Christian World*, New Haven: Yale University Press, 1983, 221–41.
3 Contrary to the hypothesis of Dieter Georgi in *Die Gegner des Paulus im zweiten Korintherbrief*, Neukirchen, 1964.
4 Aristotle, in *On the Generation of Animals*, refers in a score of passages to physiological details which are documented in the Hippocratic corpus, though without explicit reference to Hippocrates. The nearest he comes to such an identification of his worthy opponents is the mention of "certain physiologers" (δ' βούλονται λέγειν τινὲς τῶυ φυσικῶν), by which he must certainly be alluding to Hippocrates.
5 For a full and fair assessment of Galen, including the antecedents which helped to shape his views of medicine, see Owsei Temkin, *Galenism: Rise and Decline of a Medical Philosophy*, Ithaca, NY: Cornell University Press, 1973.
6 Here I am employing the methods of sociology-of-knowledge as it contributes to historical method – an approach which I have set out in my *Christian Origins in Sociological Perspective*, Philadelphia: The Westminster Press, 1980, and in *Miracle in the Early Christian World*, New Haven: Yale University Press, 1983, esp. 42–77.
7 W.W.R. Rivers, *Medicine, Magic and Religion*, London: Kegan Paul, 1924, vii.
8 Pliny the Elder, *Natural History* XXIX.7, Cambridge, Mass.: Harvard University Press; London: W. Heinemann Ltd, 1936–63.

1 Healing in the Old Testament and post-biblical traditions

1 It is unlikely that *sr't* is simply to be equated with what is now known as leprosy. Rather, it seems likely that it includes a number of curable diseases of the skin, all of which (including leprosy) were the basis for ritual ostracism in Israel under the Priestly Code.
2 Mary Douglas (in *Purity and Danger*, London: Routledge & Kegan Paul [1966] 1976) is emphatic that the ritual process aims at purification and was not regarded as a primitive medical procedure.

3 The imagery of Isa 35:1–10 is reminiscent of Isa 40, and may also come from the post-exilic period.

4 The technique of throwing a tree in the water resembles magic, but the instruction is given directly by Yahweh.

5 See pp. 72–4, 90.

6 There are direct correspondences between passages in Jeremiah and the psalms: cf. Jer 17:7–8 with Psa 1:1–3; Jer 17:10 with Psa 62:12.

7 This wady, which has water only during the rainy season, is Wady Qumran. Apparently the Dead Sea community chose this location for settlement in anticipation of the fulfilment of this prophecy.

8 Here of course Luke is dependent on the LXX, rather than on the textually, and therefore exegetically, uncertain Hebrew text.

9 Geza Vermes, *Jesus the Jew*, New York: Macmillan, 1973, 61.

10 See, for example, H. C. Kee, "The Ethical Dimensions of the Testaments of the XII as a Clue to Provenance," NTS 24 (1978), 259–70.

11 Pliny, *Natural History* XXIII.1.

12 Pliny, *Natural History* XXIX.1.

13 See below, pp. 23–5.

14 G. Vermes, *Jesus the Jew*, 61. Vermes draws attention to the factor of demons and exorcism in Tobit, but it is not relevant for his purpose to point out the wider links with medicine and with the angels in this fascinating story of healing among the Jews in exile.

15 See pp. 46–7 and Appendix.

16 In *On the Contemplative Life* 2 and *Hypothetica* 2.11–13. Another description of the Essenes appears in Philo's *Quod Omni Probus* 75–91.

17 Josephus, *Antiquities* 8.45.

18 See H. C. Kee, "The Terminology of Mark's Exorcism Stories," NTS 14 (1968), 232–46, and the further discussion in *Miracle in the Early Christian World*, 161–5.

2 Medicine in the Greek and Roman traditions

1 See the discussion of "Asklepios the Healer" in my *Miracle in the Early Christian World*, 78–103.

2 Summarized from Louis Cohn-Haft, *The Public Physician of Ancient Greece*, Northampton, Mass.: Smith College Studies in History, 1956, 11–18.

3 L. Edelstein, "Greek Medicine in its Relation to Religion and Magic", in *Ancient Medicine*, Baltimore: Johns Hopkins Press, 1967, 217–46. Reprinted from *Bulletin of the Institute for the History of Medicine* V (1937).

4 Wm Arthur Heidel, *Hippocratic Medicine: Its Spirit and Method*, New York: Columbia University Press, 1941, 12.

5 Heidel, *Hippocratic Medicine*, 13.

6 Hippocrates, *De Arte* x f. vol. VI, 16ff, Littré edition.

7 Hippocrates, *Epidemics* I, in *Hippocrates*, tr. by W. H. S. Jones, Loeb Classical Library, London: W. Heinemann Ltd; New York: G. P. Putnam's Sons, 1923.

8 Hippocrates, *Praescriptio* vi.
9 Heidel, *Hippocratic Medicine*, 130.
10 Heidel, *Hippocratic Medicine*, 134.
11 Heidel, *Hippocratic Medicine*, 136–7.
12 Heidel, *Hippocratic Medicine*, 115.
13 Heidel, *Hippocratic Medicine*, 125–6.
14 Wesley D. Smith, *The Hippocratic Tradition*, Ithaca, NY: Cornell University Press, 1979, 30.
15 Littré, following Galen, rejected as inauthentic the Hippocratic tradition *On Regimen*, but Smith believes a fragment of Menon's *History of Medicine* found in Egypt is dependent on this document, and that Galen rejected it because it did not fit his own version of the four-humour theory. See W. D. Smith, *Hippocratic Tradition*, 36–60.
16 W. D. Smith, *Hippocratic Tradition*, 77–9, 124–5.
17 W. D. Smith, *Hippocratic Tradition*, 105–45.
18 Cf., however, Luis Garcia Ballester, "Galen as a Medical Practitioner: Problems in Diagnosis", in *Galen: Problems and Prospects*, ed. by Vivian Nutton. London: Wellcome Institute of the History of Medicine, 1981: "The new feature in Galen is the insistence that scientific diagnosis be made solely on the basis of reason", 15. The twin enterprises of diagnosis and prognosis rest on θεωρία, 17.
19 P. M. Fraser, *Ptolemaic Alexandria*, 3 vols, Oxford: Clarendon Press, 1972, 348.
20 Susan M. Sherwin-White, *Ancient Cos*. Hypomnemata: Untersuchungen zur Antike und zu ihrem Nachleben. Heft 51. Göttingen: Vandenhoeck and Ruprecht, 1978, 257.
21 S. M. Sherwin-White, *Ancient Cos*, 275.
22 L. Cohn-Haft, *Public Physician*, 27.
23 S. Sherwin-White, *Ancient Cos*, 288–9.
24 P. M. Fraser, *Ptolemaic Alexandria*, 342.
25 G. E. R. Lloyd, *Greek Science After Aristotle*. London: Chatto and Windus, 1973, 89.
26 G. E. R. Lloyd, *Greek Science After Aristotle*, 88. Also P. M. Fraser, *Ptolemaic Alexandria*, 350–1.
27 P. M. Fraser, *Ptolemaic Alexandria*, 354–5.
28 Herophilus the Sophist, in *Notices et Extraits des Manuscrits de la Bibliothèque du Roi*, ed. by M. Boissonade, vol. 11, pt 2. Paris: Imprimerie Royale, 1827, 178–273. The text is also available in *Physici et Medici Graeci Minores*, vol. 2, ed. by J. L. Ideler (1841). Repr. Amsterdam: Hakkert, 1963, 409–17.
29 In his notes to the section of the text dealing with January, Boissonade discusses at great length the problem of the names of the constellations, and reports on consultations he has had with others about the identity of such constellations as *Panthnetaion, Heliotrope and Chelidon*, 210–14.
30 P. M. Fraser, *Ptolemaic Alexandria*, 361–2.
31 John Scarborough, *Roman Medicine*, Ithaca: Cornell University Press (1969), 1976, 15–16.

32 According to Livy (*From the Founding of the City*, tr. by R.O. Foster, Loeb Classical Library, London: W. Heinemann Ltd; New York: G.P. Putnam's Sons, 1922, 10:47, 11) the oracles were apparently from the Sibyllines; according to Ovid (*Metamorphoses*, tr. with an Intro. by Mary M. Innes, Baltimore: Penguin Books, 1973, 19:625—744) it was the Delphic oracle which thus counselled.

33 John Scarborough, *Roman Medicine*, 74.

34 John Scarborough, *Roman Medicine*, 66—70.

35 Varro I.12.

36 Columella I.5.

37 See J. Scarborough, *Roman Medicine*, Pl. 18 and fig. 7—9.

38 Celsus, *De Medicina*, tr. by W.G. Spencer, Loeb Classical Library, London: W. Heinemann Ltd, Cambridge, Mass.: Harvard University Press, 1935—8 vol. I, Prooemium 9—13.

39 Celsus, *De Medicina* I, LCL 24—6. On the four elements of Empedocles, cf. Plato, *Timaeus*, 82 and Hippocrates IV. The theorists were by no means of one mind in their attempts to show correspondences between the four elements and the humours.

40 Celsus, *De Medicina* I, LCL 41. All subsequent references in parentheses are to Celsus, with the book indicated by the Roman numeral.

41 This practice consisted of placing a cup over an incision made in the body (anywhere, frequently the skull), on the assumption that the supposed vacuum in the empty cup would draw out the sickness substance.

42 W.G. Spencer, in introduction to volume II of Celsus, *De Medicina* in LCL, London: W. Heinemann Ltd, 1958, ix.

43 The standard edition of Dioscorides is *De Materia Medica*, Bk 5, ed. by Max Wellman (1908), Berlin: Weidmannsche Verlagsbuchhandlung, repr. 1958. There is a seventeenth-century English translation by John Goodyer, ed. by R.T. Gunther, in *Dioscorides: Greek Herbal* (1934), New York: Hafner, (1959), 1968.

44 Rufus of Ephesus, *Oeuvres*, ed. and tr. by C. Daremberg and C.E. Ruelle, repr. Amsterdam, 1963.

45 Rufus von Ephesos, *Krankenjournale*, ed. and tr. by Manfred Ullmann, Wiesbaden: Harrasowitz, 1978.

46 See *Rufus*, ed. by Ullmann, where the balancing of the temperaments is also discussed in III.7; IV.4; V.5.

47 Included in the older corpus ed. by Daremberg (note 44), and in two edns by Hans Gärtner, *Corpus Medicorum Graecorum*, Suppl. IX Berlin: Akademie Verlag, 1962 and *Quaestiones Medicales*, Leipzig: Teubner, 1970.

48 Rufus, *Corpus* 13.72—3.

49 *Rufus von Ephesos: Über die Nieren- und Blasenleiden*, ed. Alexander Sideras. In *Corpus Medicorum Graecorum* III.1 1977, 9.8—12.

50 Daremberg, ed., *Oeuvres, On Satyriasis and Gonorrhoea*.

51 Rufus von Ephesos, *Krankenjournale*, ed. and tr. by Manfred Ullmann, II (68—72, in my translation).

52 The authenticity of these treatises attributed to Rufus has been questioned, but they fit well with the rest of the corpus of Rufus' works.
53 G. W. Bowersock, *Greek Sophists in the Roman Empire*: Oxford: Clarendon Press, 1969, 59–60.
54 Bowersock, *Sophists*, 59.
55 Bowersock, *Sophists*, 66.
56 Owsei Temkin, *Galenism: Rise and Decline of a Medical Philosophy*, 1973, 5, 11, 17.
57 Wesley D. Smith, *Hippocratic Tradition*, 30.
58 Ballester, "Galen as Medical Practitioner", 20.
59 Ballester, "Galen as Medical Practitioner", 35.
60 Galen, *On Anatomical Procedures*, Intro. and tr. by Charles Singer, London: Wellcome Museum of History of Medicine, 1956.
61 Galen, *On Medical Experience*, tr. from the Arabic by R. Walger, Oxford: Oxford University Press, 1944.
62 Rudolph E. Siegel, *Galen's System of Physiology and Medicine: An Analysis of his Doctrines and Observations on Bloodflow, Respiration, Humans and Internal Diseases*, Basel and New York: S. Karger, 1968.
63 Siegel, *Physiology*, 29.
64 Siegel, *Physiology*, 86–7.
65 Siegel, *Physiology*, 101–4.
66 Siegel, *Physiology*, 125.
67 Siegel, *Physiology*, 184–90.
68 Siegel, *Physiology*, 196–201.
69 Siegel, *Physiology*, 216–322.
70 Siegel, *Physiology*, 352–9.
71 Siegel, *Physiology*, 360–1.
72 Described by Wesley D. Smith, *Hippocratic Tradition*, 63.
73 G. W. Bowersock, *Greek Sophists*, 69. Complete list of Asklepia in J. Scarborough, W. 51 p. 222.
74 L. and E. J. Edelstein, *Asclepius Testimonies* vol. I, Baltimore: John Hopkins, 1945, T 473.
75 O. Temkin, *Galenism*, 24.
76 *Adhortatio ad Artes Addiscendas*, Eng tr. by Joseph Walsh, "Galen's Exhortation to the Study of the Arts, Especially Medicine", *Medical Life* 37 (1930), 507–29.
77 Temkin, *Galenism*, 27.
78 Fridolf Kudlien, "Galen's Religious Beliefs", in *Galen: Problems and Prospects*, ed. by Vivian Nutton, London: Wellcome Institute of History of Medicine, 1981, 119–21.
79 Kudlien, "Galen's Religious Beliefs", 122.
80 Kudlien, "Galen's Religious Beliefs", 123–4.
81 L. Edelstein, "Greek Medicine", 246.
82 This is proposed by Christian Habicht, *Die Inschriften des Asklepions* (in Altertümer von Pergamon, Bd 8.3 Deutsches Archäologisches Institut), Berlin: W. de Gruyter, 1969. The refutation in F. Kudlien, "Galen's Religious Beliefs", 121.

83 F. Kundlien, "Galen's Religious Beliefs", 126–7. The material from Galen is in *De lib. prop.* 2:xix.19; *De sent.* 2.4; *Asklepios Testimonies* 458.

84 L. Edelstein, "Greek Medicine", 217.

85 L. Edelstein, "Greek Medicine", 218.

86 L. Edelstein, "Greek Medicine", 246.

87 L. Edelstein, "Greek Medicine", 231. Also in J. Scarborough, *Roman Medicine*, 120.

88 Galen, *Opera Omnia*, ed. by C. G. Kuhn. Repr. Hildesheim, 20 vols. IX.910–913.

89 Galen, *Opera Omnia*, XV.313–16.

90 Dio Chrysostom, *Discourses* XXXIII.6 – LCL III, tr. by J. W. Cohoon and H. Lamar Crosby, London: W. Heinemann Ltd, 1961–4, 279.

91 J. Scarborough, *Roman Medicine*, 108.

92 See the careful analysis and negative results of Henry J. Cadbury's classic study of the so-called medical language of Luke in *The Style and Literary Method of Luke*, Cambridge, Mass.: Harvard University Press, 1920.

93 Cf. R. Bultmann, *History of Synoptic Tradition*, 209–15, 239–44. Cf. M. Dibelius, *From Tradition to Gospel*, Eng. tr. by B. L. Woolf, New York: Charles Scribner's Sons, n.d.

3 Miracle

1 The background and development of the devotion to Isis in the early Roman period is traced in my *Miracle in the Early Christian World*, 105–45.

2 Text in Yves Grandjean, *Une Nouvelle Arétalogie d'Isis à Maroneé*, Leiden: Brill, 1975.

3 Diodorus Siculus, *Library of History* tr. by John Skelton, Oxford: Oxford University Press, 1956–7, 1.25.3.

4 Diodorus Siculus, *Library of History* 1.25.5.

5 Aristophanes, *Plautus*, in *Comedies of Aristophanes*, London: printed by A. J. Valpy for Lackington, Allen, 1812, Act 3, scene 2. Details of this and other aspects of the Asklepios cult in H. C. Kee, *Miracle in the Early Christian World*, ch. 3, "Asklepios the Healer", 78–104.

6 Livy, *From the Founding of the City*, 10:47; 11.

7 Ovid, *Metamorphoses*, 15.625–744.

8 Quoted from H. C. Kee, *Miracle in the Early Christian World*, 85.

9 In H. C. Kee, *Community of the New Age*, Macon, Ga: Macon University Press, 2nd edn, 1984, 79–87.

10 Basic studies of community definition are those of Mary Douglas, *Purity and Danger*, London: Routledge and Kegan Paul, 1966, 1976, and *Natural Symbols: Explorations in Cosmology*, New York: Random House, 1970, 1973, and Hans J. Mol, *Identity and the Sacred*, New York: Free Press, 1977. A programmatic study of the implications of these methods for the study of early Christianity

is H.C. Kee, *Christian Origins in Sociological Perspective*, Philadelphia: Westminster Press, 1980. A direct application of these methods to the study of our period is that of Goran Forkman, *The Limits of the Religious Community: Expulsion from the Religious Community within the Qumran Sect, within Rabbinic Judaism, and within Primitive Christianity*, Lund: C.W.K. Gleerup, 1972.

11 Dibelius, *From Tradition to Gospel*, 91–3.
12 Dibelius, *From Tradition to Gospel*, 99.
13 Dibelius, *From Tradition to Gospel*, 100–1.
14 Rudolf Bultmann, *History of the Synoptic Tradition*, tr. by John Marsh. New York, Harper and Row, 1963, 240–1.
15 Dibelius, *From Tradition to Gospel*, 102.
16 Geza Vermes, *Jesus the Jew*, New York: Macmillan, 1973.
17 Vermes, *Jesus the Jew*, 20–6, 58–82.
18 Examples of Harnack's scholarly researches include Adolf von Harnack, *Geschichte der altchristlichen Literatur*, Leipzig, 1897–1904; *The Mission and Expansion of Christianity*, New York: Putnam, 1908; *Outlines of Dogma*, Eng. ed. Boston: Beacon Press, 1959.
19 Adolf von Harnack, *What is Christianity?* New York: Putnam, 1901. The more precise and revealing title of the German original, *Das Wesen Christentums* was altered in the English translation to the interrogative form, *What is Christianity?*
20 Rudolf Bultmann, *Jesus* (1926) Tubingen: Mohr 1951. The English translation is *Jesus and the Word*, tr. by L.P. Smith and E.H. Lantero, New York: Scribner, 1934.
21 Dibelius, *From Tradition to Gospel*, 80–4; it is suggested that traces of thaumaturgic technique, including diagnoses of the illness of those about to be healed, have been imported by the tradition from Hellenistic sources.
22 On the theory that Jesus was a magician (or the variant notion that the gospel writers portray him as such) see Chapter 4.
23 The classic examination of the element of miracle in the rabbinic tradition is by Paul Fiebig, *Die jüdische Wundergeschichten*. Tübingen: Mohr, 1911. See the discussion below, pp.80–3, of Geza Vermes' more recent, historical reconstruction of rabbinical practice in healing and exorcisms, in *Jesus the Jew*.
24 Fiebig, *Wundergeschichten*, 1–28.
25 Vermes, *Jesus the Jew*, 19.
26 Vermes, *Jesus the Jew*, 28.
27 Vermes, *Jesus the Jew*, 26.
28 Vermes, *Jesus the Jew*, 37.
29 Vermes, *Jesus the Jew*, 64.
30 Summarized in Kee, *Miracle in the Early Christian World*, 178–9.
31 Vermes, *Jesus the Jew*, 74–5, where references are given to Hanina in the rabbinic material: yBer 9a; tBer 2:20; bBer 33a.
32 Vermes, *Jesus the Jew*, 58–82.
33 Jacob Neusner, *A History of the Jews in Babylon*, vol.IV, *The Age of Shapur III (307–309 C.E.)*, 362.

34 Cf. Dio Cassius 61:35; 63.185.235.
35 Suetonius, *The Twelve Caesars* (Vespasian) tr. by Robert Graves, Harmondsworth, Middlesex; Baltimore: Penguin Books, 1957, 5.6.
36 Tacitus, *Histories*, tr. by G. G. Ramsay, London: J. Murray, 1915, 4.lxxxig 4.lxxvii.
37 Typical of the older form critical reconstruction of the gospel tradition is the theory expressed by Karl Kundsin (in *Form Criticism*, tr. by F. C. Grant, New York: Harper, 1934, 1962, 99) that both the apocalyptic eschatology attributed to Jesus in the gospels and his miracle working are part of the "pre-Christian and sub-Christian" ideas which permeated the early Christian communities under the influence of Jewish and Hellenistic speculation respectively (100). It was Mark, Kundsin declared, who for the first time put together all the narratives of the miracles of Jesus, thereby putting him in the class with Hellenistic wonder-workers and epiphanic divine figures from the Hellenistic religious traditions (123). H. D. Betz, in his article on *Gottmensch* in the *Reallexicon für Antike und Christentum* (Stuttgart, 1982), after tracing the application of the title θεῖος ἀνήρ to healers, philosophers, seers and oracles in the Hellenistic period, offers the generalization that the term is used of a philosopher by whose philosophical and ethical knowledge he is able to perform miracles. The prime example he offers is Apollonius of Tyana as described by Philostratus (Col. 248–51). He describes Mark, after having traced the development of the Pauline Christology and its use of the concept, as having completely reworked the material that came to him, placing the story of Jesus in an historical context, and depicting him as a divine being who chose to suffer death, which occurs as the "ultimate epiphany of the divine man" (301–2). Why suffering and death would be the "ultimate" self-disclosure of a miracle-working philosopher type is not readily apparent from Betz' presentation.
38 Two detailed studies of the "divine man" are those by David L. Tiede (*The Charismatic Figure as Miracle Worker*, SBLDS 1. Missoula, Mont., 1972) and by Carl Holladay (*Theios Aner in Hellenistic Judaism*, SBLDS 40. Missoula, Mont., 1977). Tiede has demonstrated the range of ways in which the term was used in the Graeco-Roman period, and how it shifted from an earlier emphasis on the wise man to the shaman, for which Pythagoras was the model. Holladay has concentrated on Philo of Alexandria and Josephus, for whom the model was that of a virtuous wise man. The *theios aner* stands in special relationship to God by virtue of insight and leadership role, for which Moses is the ideal type, but there is never any notion of divinization of such a figure, nor does the performance of miracle constitute a significant factor. To represent miracle-working as a central feature of the role of the divine man or as the clue to his divine relationship has no basis in the first-century evidence.
39 T. Weeden, *Mark: Traditions in Conflict*. Philadelphia, 1971.
40 Philostratus, *Life of Apollonius of Tyana*, tr. by Charles P. Eeels, New York: AMS Press, 1967, 4.16; 6.11; 8.7.

41 Philostratus, *Life of Apollonius*, 7.14–15; 2.14; 5.36; 6.29.
42 The direct reference to Diogenes and Crates, in addition to Apollonius' adopting the life of poverty and utter simplicity, make this evident.
43 Philostratus, *Life of Apollonius*, 2.29, 40; 3.28; 5.27–35.
44 Philostratus, *Life of Apollonius*, 1.19.
45 Philostratus, *Life of Apollonius*, 5.11, 18, 35; 6.32; 3.12.
46 Philostratus, *Life of Apollonius*, 2.37; 3.42.
47 Philostratus, *Life of Apollonius*, 1.19.
48 Philostratus, *Life of Apollonius*, 4.45.
49 Philostratus, *Life of Apollonius*, 4.3.
50 Philostratus, *Life of Apollonius*, 8.7.
51 Philostratus, *Life of Apollonius*, 3.38.
52 Philostratus, *Life of Apollonius*, 6.42.
53 Philostratus, *Life of Apollonius*, 8.7.
54 See my discussion of symbolization in *Miracle in the Early Christian World*, 232–4, which builds on insights from Suzanne Langer, *Philosophy in a New Key: A Study in the Symbolism of Rite and Act*, Cambridge, Mass.: Harvard University Press, 1942, 1957, 1976.
55 Langer, *Philosophy*, 30.
56 Langer, *Philosophy*, 45, 97.
57 Robert J. Lifton, *The Broken Connection*, New York: Simon and Schuster, 1979, 283.
58 R. J. Lifton, *Broken Connection*, 284.
59 Plutarch, *De Iside*, tr. by J. G. Griffiths, Cardiff: University of Wales Press, 1970, 20.
60 Plutarch, *De Iside*, 65–6.
61 Plutarch, *De Iside*, 72.
62 Plutarch, *De Iside*, 67, 75.
63 Plutarch, *De Iside*, 78.
64 Plutarch, *De Iside*, 3.
65 Plutarch, *De Iside*, 3.
66 Aelius Aristides, *Sacred Discourses*, ed. and tr. by C. A. Behr, LCL, Cambridge, Mass.: Harvard University Press, 1973.
67 Aelius Aristides, *In Defense of Oratory*, tr. by C. A. Behr, Cambridge, Mass.: Harvard University Press, 1973. Roman numerals = sections, arabic numerals = line.
68 Aelius Aristides, *In Defense of Oratory*, 149–56.

4 Magic

1 For details, see my *Miracle in the Early Christian World*, 134–9.
2 *The Apologia and Florida of Apuleius of Madaura*, Intro. and tr. by H. E. Butler, Oxford: Clarendon Press, 1909.
3 Apuleius, *Apologia*, Introduction, "That Apuleius was acquitted cannot be doubted", 11.
4 Apuleius, *Apologia*, Ch., 47.
5 Herodotus. I.32.

6 E. M. Butler, *The Myth of the Magus*, Cambridge: Cambridge University Press, 1948, 20–2.

7 E. M. Butler, *Ritual Magic*, Cambridge: Cambridge Univesity Press, 1949, 19.

8 A. D. Nock, "Paul and the Magus" in *Beginnings of Christianity* V, ed. by F. J. Foakes-Jackson and K. Lake, Grand Rapids, Baker, Mich. 1933, 1966 repr., 164–88.

9 Nock, "Paul and the Magus," 171.

10 Nock, "Paul and the Magus," 179–81.

11 Nock, "Paul and the Magus," 164, 173.

12 Classic studies of magic include Bronislaw Malinowski, *Magic, Science and Religion*, Garden City, NY: Doubleday (1948) 1954; M. Mauss, *A General Theory of Magic*, New York: Norton, 1972. Discussions of magic in a broad anthropological context include Lucy Mair, *An Introduction to Social Anthropology*, Oxford: Clarendon Press, 1972, 225–9.

13 Richard Cavendish, *A History of Magic*, London: Weidenfeld and Nicolson, 1977, 13.

14 *Papyri Graecae Magicae: Die griechische Zauberpapyri*, ed. by Karl Preisendanz; 2nd edn, Albert Henrichs, Stuttgart: Teubner, 1973.

15 Here the insights of sociology-of-knowledge are of paramount importance. See my discussion of this factor and its significance for historical interpretation in *Miracle in the Early Christian World*, esp. Ch. 2, "Personal Identity and World Construction", and in *Christian Origins in Sociological Perspective*.

16 On magical knots, Cyrus L. Day, *Quipus and Witches' Knots: The Role of the Knot in Primitive and Ancient Cultures*, Lawrence, Kansas: University of Kansas Press, 1967.

17 Peter Brown, "Sorcery, Demons and the Rise of Christianity", in *Religion and Society in the Age of St. Augustine*. New York: Harper and Row, 1972, 120–1.

18 Morton Smith, *Jesus the Magician*, New York: Harper and Row, 1978; John M. Hull, *Hellenistic Magic and the Synoptic Tradition*. London: SCM, 1974.

19 Morton Smith, *Jesus the Magician*, 107.

20 Morton Smith, *Jesus the Magician*, 114.

21 Morton Smith, *Jesus the Magician*, 123.

22 Morton Smith, *Jesus the Magician*, 123.

23 Morton Smith, *Jesus the Magician*, 137.

24 Morton Smith, *Jesus the Magician*, 137–8.

25 John M. Hull, *Hellenistic Magic and the Synoptic Tradition*, London: SCM Press, 1967 (SBT, 2nd series 28), 48.

26 John M. Hull, *Hellenistic Magic*, 37–8.

27 John M. Hull, *Hellenistic Magic*, 57.

28 Peter Brown, "Sorcery, Demons and the Rise of Christianity", 119–46.

29 John Ferguson, *The Religions of the Roman Empire*, Ithaca, NY: Cornell University Press, 1970.

30 E. R. Dodds, *Pagan and Christian in an Age of Anxiety*, New York: Norton, 1965, 124–5.
31 Origen, *Contra Celsum*, tr. H. Chadwick, Cambridge: Cambridge University Press, 1965.
32 Carl Andresen, *Logos und Nomos: Die Polemik Kelsos wider das Urchristentum*, Berlin: Walter de Gruyter, 1955.
33 Cambridge, Mass.: The Philadelphia Patristics Foundation, 1983.
34 Chico, Calif.: Scholars Press, 1981.
35 New Haven: Yale University Press, 1984.
36 R. Wilken, *Christians as the Romans Saw Them*, New Haven: Yale University Press, 1984, 120–5.
37 See my *Miracle in the Early Christian World*, 183–90.

5 Concluding Observations

1 E. R. Dodds, *Pagan and Christian in an Age of Anxiety*, 124–5.
2 *Galenus Opera Omnia*, ed. Kuhn, XI. 792.
3 Edelstein, L., "Greek Medicine in its Relation to Religion and Magic", London: *Bulletin of the Institute of the History of Medicine* V. 1937, 227.
4 H. C. Kee, *Jesus in History*, New York: Harcourt, Brace, Jovanovich, 2nd edn, 1977, 177–84.

Appendix

1 Allegro, *Myth*, 235–6.
2 For a study of these scripts see F. M. Cross, "The Development of the Jewish Scripts", in *The Bible and the Ancient Near East: Essays in Honor of William Foxwell Albright*, ed. G. E. Wright (Anchor Books, A431. Garden City, NY: Doubleday, 1965) pp. 170–264, esp. p. 139.
3 The degree of certainty of a reading is indicated according to the standard methodology explained in D. Barthélemy and J. T. Milik (editors), *Qumran Cave I* (Discoveries in the Judean Desert 1; Oxford: Clarendon Press, 1955) pp. 46–8. I wish to thank Professor E. Qimron for helping me improve the transcription.
4 The text is written *scriptio continua*, and *Petros* is separated on two lines. Both phenomena are otiose.
5 See my preliminary comments in *The Discovery of a Dead Sea Scroll (4Q Therapeia): Its Importance in the History of Medicine and Jesus Research* (Lubbock, Texas: I ASALS, 1985).

BIBLIOGRAPHY

Primary Sources in Translation

Aelius Aristides, *In Defense of Oratory*, tr. by C.A. Behr, Loeb Classical Library, Cambridge, Mass.: Harvard University Press, 1973.
  Sacred Discourses, tr. by C.A. Behr, Loeb Classical Library, Cambridge, Mass.: Harvard University Press, 1973.
Apuleius, Lucius, *Metamorphoses*, tr. by W. Adlington (1566), rev. by S. Gaselee, London: W. Heinemann Ltd; New York, G.P. Putnam's Sons, 1924.
  The Apologia and Florida of Apuleius of Madaura, intro, and tr. by H.E. Butler. Oxford: Clarendon Press, 1909.
Aristophanes, *Plutus*, in *Comedies of Aristophanes*, London: printed by A.J. Valpy for Lackington, Allen, 1812.
Aristotle, *On the Generation of Animals*, tr. by A.L. Peck, Loeb Classical Library, Cambridge, Mass.: Harvard University Press; London: W. Heinemann Ltd, 1943.
Celsus, *De Medicina*, tr. by W.G. Spencer, Loeb Classical Library, London: W. Heinemann Ltd; Cambridge, Mass.: Harvard University Press, 1935–8.
Cicero, *Laws (De Legibus)*, tr. by C.W. Keyes, Loeb Classical Library, London: W. Heinemann Ltd; Cambridge, Mass.: Harvard University Press, 1951, 1972.
  On the Nature of the Gods, tr. by Horace C.P. Macgregor, Harmondsworth: Penguin, 1972.
Dio Cassius, *Roman History*, tr. by Earnest Cary, 9 vols., London: W. Heinemann Ltd; New York: Macmillan Co., 1914–27.
Dio Chrysostom, *Discourses*, 5 vols., tr. by J.W. Cohoon and H. Lamar Crosby, London: W. Heinemann Ltd, 1961–4.
Diodorus Siculus, *Bibliotheca historia* (Library of History), tr. by John Skelton, Oxford: Oxford University Press, 1956–7.
Dioscorides, *Greek Herbal*, Eng. tr. by John Goodyer, ed. by R.T. Gunther, in *Dioscorides: Greek Herbal* (1934), New York: Hafner (1959), 1968. Cf. also *De Materia Medica*, Bk 5, ed. by Max Wellman (1908), Berlin: Weidmannsche Verlagsbuchhandlung, repr. 1958.
Galenus opera omnia, ed. by C.G. Kuhn, repr. Hildesheim, 20 vols.
Galen, *Adhortatio ad Artes Addiscendas*, tr. by Joseph Walsh, "Galen's Exhortation to the Study of the Arts, Especially Medicine", *Medical Life* 37 (1930), 507–29.

On Anatomical Procedures, intro. and tr. by Charles Singer, London: Wellcome Museum of History of Medicine, 1956.

On Medical Experiences, tr. by R. Walger, Oxford: Oxford University Press, 1944.

Genesis Apocryphon, in *The Dead Sea Scrolls in English*, ed. by Geza Vermes, Baltimore: Penguin Books, 1962.

Herophilus the Sophist, in *Notices et Extraits des Manuscrits de la Bibliothèque du Roi*, ed. by M. Boissonade, vol. 11, pt 2, Paris: Imprimerie Royale, 1827. The text is also available in *Physici et Medici Graeci Minores*, vol. 2, ed. by J. L. Ideler (1841), repr. Amsterdam: Hakkert, 1963, 409–17.

Hippocrates, tr. by W. H. S. Jones, Loeb Classical Library, London: W. Heinemann Ltd; New York: G. P. Putnam's Sons, 1923.

Concerning Airs, vol. 1, 71–117.

Epidemics I, vol. 1, 146–211.

Precepts, vol. 1, 313–33.

On Regimen, vol. 2, 57–126.

The Art, vol. 2, 185–218.

On Regimen in Acute Diseases, xxxviii–lv, 224–447.

Oeuvres complètes, Littré edition, 10 vols, Paris, 1839–61.

De decenti habitu, iv, vol. lx.

Homer, *The Iliad*, tr. by E. V. Rieu, Baltimore: Penguin Books, 1973, *ca* 1950.

The Odyssey, tr. by Ennis Rees, Indianapolis: Bobbs-Merrill Educational Pub., *c.* 1977.

Livy, *From the Founding of the City*, tr. by R. O. Foster, Loeb Classical Library, London: W. Heinemann Ltd; New York: G. P. Putnam's Sons, 1922.

Lucian, *Alexander the False Prophet*, tr. by A. Harmon, Loeb Classical Library, vol. IV, London: W. Heinemann Ltd, 1961.

Lexiphanes, tr. by A. M. Harmon, Loeb Classical Library, vol. V, London: W. Heinemann Ltd, 1962.

The Parliament of the Gods, tr. by A. M. Harmon, Loeb Classical Library, vol. V, London: W. Heinemann Ltd, 1962.

The Passing of Peregrinus, tr. by A. M. Harmon, Loeb Classical Library, vol. V, London: W. Heinemann Ltd; 1962.

Origen, *Contra Celsum*, tr. with an intro. and notes by Henry Chadwick, Cambridge: Cambridge University Press, 1965.

Ovid, *Metamorphoses*, tr. with an intro. by Mary M. Innes, Baltimore: Penguin Books, 1973.

Papyri Graecae Magicae: Die griechische Zauberpapyri, ed. by Karl Preisendanz; 2nd edn, Albert Henrichs, Stuttgart: Teubner, 1973.

Philostratus, *Life of Apollonius of Tyana*, tr. by Charles P. Eells, New York: AMS Press, 1967.

Pindar, *Pythian Ode* III, 47–53, in *Olympian and Pythian Odes*, ed. by Basil Gildersleeve, St Claire Shores, Miss.: Scholarly Press, 1970.

Plato, *Alcibiades*, tr. and comm. by William O'Neill, The Hague: M. Nijhoff, 1971.

Gorgias 465a, tr. with notes by Terrence Irwin, Oxford: Clarendon Press, 1979.

Laws 902c, ed. and intro. by E. B. England, New York: Arno Press, 1976.
Phaedrus 270d ff. (along with the seventh and eighth letters), tr. with an intro. by Walter Hamilton, Harmondsworth: Penguin Books, 1973.
The Republic, tr. by G. M. A. Grube, Indianapolis: Hackett Publ. Co., 1974.
Timaeus, tr. with an intro. by H. D. D. Lee, Baltimore: Penguin Books, 1965.
Pliny the Elder, *Natural History*, with Engl. tr. by H. Rackham, Cambridge, Mass.: Harvard University Press; London: W. Heinemann Ltd, 1936–63, 10 vols.
Plutarch, *De Iside*, tr. by J. G. Griffiths, Cardiff: University of Wales Press, 1970. (Title of work, *De Iside et Osiride*.)
"Lycurgus of Numa", *Lives, Vol.*1, Loeb Classical Library, London: W. Heinemann Ltd (1914), 1983.
Rufus, *Concerning the Interrogation of the Sick*, in Rufus, *Krankenjournale* III.1. Berlin: Akademie Verlag, 1979, and in Hans Gärtner, *Corpus Medicorum Graecorum*, Supp. IX, Berlin: Akademie Verlag, 1962, and *Quaestiones Medicales*. Leipzig: Teubner, 1970.
Rufus of Ephesus, *Oeuvres*, ed. and French tr. by C. Daremberg and C. E. Ruelle, repr. Amsterdam, 1963. Also Rufus von Ephesus, *Krankenjournale*, ed. and tr. by Manfred Ullmann, Wiesbaden: Harrasowitz, 1978. Eng. tr. of title, *Journal of the Sick*.
Rufus von Ephesos: *Uber die Nieren-und Blasenleiden*, ed. Alexander Sideras. In *Corpus Medicorum Graecorum* III.1, 1977.
Suetonius, *The Twelve Caesars* (Vespasian, 5.6) tr. by Robert Graves, Harmondsworth: Penguin Books, 1957.
Tacitus, *Histories*, tr. by G. G. Ramsay, London: J. Murray, 1915.
Testaments of the Twelve Patriarchs and *I Enoch*, both in *The Old Testament Pseudepigraph*, ed. by James H. Charlesworth, vol. 1, Garden City, NY: Doubleday, 1983.
4Q Therapeia. See appendix of present work.

Secondary Sources

Allegro, J. M., *The Dead Sea Scrolls and the Christian Myth*, Newton Abbot: Westbridge Books, 1979; repr. New York: Promtheus Books, 1984.
Andresen, Carl, *Logos und Nomos: Die Polemik Kelsos wider das Urchristentum*, Berlin: Walter de Gruyter, 1955.
Ballester, Luis Garcia, "Galen as a Medical Practitioner: Problems in Diagnosis", in *Galen: Problems and Prospects*, ed. by Vivian Nutton, London: Wellcome Institute of the History of Medicine, 1981.
Barthélemy, D., and Milik, J. T., *Qumran Cave I* (Discoveries in the Judean Desert I) Oxford: Clarendon Press, 1955, 46–8.
Bowersock, G. W., *Greek Sophists in the Roman Empire*, Oxford: Clarendon Press, 1969.
Brown, Peter, "Sorcery, Demons and the Rise of Christianity", in *Religion and Society in the Age of St. Augustine*, New York: Harper and Row, 1972.

Bultmann, Rudolf, *History of the Synoptic Tradition*, tr. by John Marsh, New York: Harper and Row, 1963, 209–15, 239–44.
Jesus and the Word, tr. by L. P. Smith and E. H. Lantero, New York: Scribner, 1934.
Butler, E. M., *Ritual Magic*, Cambridge: Cambridge University Press, 1949.
The Myth of the Magus, Cambridge: Cambridge University Press, 1948.
Cadbury, Henry J., *The Style and Literary Method of Luke*, Cambridge, Mass.: Harvard University Press, 1920.
Cavendish, Richard, *A History of Magic*, London: Weidenfeld and Nicolson, 1977.
Cohn-Haft, Louis, *The Public Physician of Ancient Greece*, Northampton, Mass.: Smith College Studies in History, 1956.
Cross, F. M., "The Development of the Jewish Scripts", in *The Bible and the Ancient Near East: Essays in Honor of William Foxwell Albright*, ed. by G. E. Wright, Anchor Books A431, Garden City, NY: Doubleday, 1965, 170–264.
Day, Cyrus L., *Quipus and Witches' Knots: The Role of the Knot in Primitive and Ancient Cultures*, Lawrence, Kansas: University of Kansas Press, 1967.
Dibelius, Martin, *From Tradition to Gospel*, tr. by B. L. Woolf, New York: Charles Scribner's Sons, n.d.
Dodds, E. R., *Pagan and Christian in an Age of Anxiety*, NY: Norton, 1965.
Douglas, Mary, *Purity and Danger*, London: Routledge & Kegan Paul, 1966.
Edelstein, L., "Greek Medicine in its Relation to Religion and Magic", in *Ancient Medicine*, Baltimore: Johns Hopkins Press, 1967, 217–46. Repr. from *Bulletin of the Institute for the History of Medicine* V (1937).
Edelstein, L. and E. J., *Asclepius Testimonies* vol. 1, Baltimore: John Hopkins Press, 1945.
Ferguson, John, *The Religions of the Roman Empire*, Ithaca: Cornell University Press, 1970.
Fiebig, Paul, *Die jüdische Wundergeschichten*, Tübingen: Mohr, 1911.
Forkmann, Goran, *The Limits of the Religious Community: Expulsion from the Religious Community within the Qumran Sect within Rabbinic Judaism, and within Primitive Christianity*, Lund: C. W. K. Gleerup, 1972.
Fraser, P. M., *Ptolemaic Alexandria*, 3 vols., Oxford: Clarendon Press, 1972.
Gallagher, Eugene V., *Divine Man or Magician? Celsus and Origen on Jesus*, Chico, Calif.: Scholars Press, 1981.
Grandjean, Yves, *Une Nouvelle Arétalogie d'Isis à Maronée*, Leiden: Brill, 1975.
Habicht, Christian, *Die Inschriften des Asklepions* (in Altertumen von Pergamon, Bd 8.3 Deutsches Archäologisches Institut), Berlin: W. de Gruyter, 1969.
Harnack, Adolf von, *What is Christianity?* New York: Putnam, 1901.
Heidel, Wm Arthur, *Hippocratic Medicine: Its Spirit and Method*, NY: Columbia University Press, 1941.
Hull, John M., *Hellenistic Magic and the Synoptic Tradition*, London: SCM Press, 1974.

Kee, Howard Clark, *Christian Origins in Sociological Perspective*, Philadelphia: The Westminster Press, 1980.
Community of the New Age, Macon, Ga: Macon University Press, 2nd edn, 1984.
Jesus in History, New York: Harcourt, Brace, Jovanovich, 2nd edn, 1977.
Miracle in the Early Christian World, New Haven: Yale University Press, 1983.
"The Ethical Dimensions of the Testaments of the XII as a Clue to Provenance," NTS 24 (1978) 259–70.
"The Terminology of Mark's Exorcism Stories," NTS 14, 1968.
Kudlien, Fridolf, "Galen's Religious Beliefs", in *Galen: Problems and Prospects*, ed. by Vivian Nutton, London: Wellcome Institute of History of Medicine, 1981.
Langer, Suzanne, *Philosophy in a New Key: A Study in the Symbolism of Rite and Act*, Cambridge, Mass.: Harvard University Press, 1942, 1957, 1976.
Lifton, Robert J., *The Broken Connection*, NY: Simon and Schuster, 1979.
Lloyd, G. E. R., *Greek Science After Aristotle*, London: Chatto and Windus, 1973.
Mair, Lucy, *An Introduction to Social Anthropology*, Oxford: Clarendon Press, 1972, 225–9.
Malinowski, Bronislaw, *Magic, Science and Religion*, Garden City, NY: Doubleday, (1948) 1954.
Mauss, M., *A General Theory of Magic*, NY: Norton, 1972.
Mol, Hans J., *Identity and the Sacred*, New York: Free Press, 1977.
Neusner, Jacob, *A History of the Jews in Babylon*, vol. IV, *The Age of Shapur, II (307–309 C.E.)*.
Nock, A. D., "Paul and the Magus" in *The Beginnings of Christianity* V., ed. by F. J. Foakes-Jackson and K. Lake, Grand Rapids Mich.: Baker, 1930, 1966 repr., 164–88.
Remus, Harold, *Pagan–Christian Conflict over Miracle in the Second Century*, Cambridge, Mass.: The Philadelphia Patristic Foundation, 1983.
Rivers, W. H. R., *Medicine, Magic and Religion*, London: Kegan Paul, 1924.
Scarborough, John, *Roman Medicine*, Ithaca, NY: Cornell University Press (1969), 1976.
Sherwin-White, Susan M., *Ancient Cos*, Hypomnemata: Untersuchungen zur Antike und zu ihrem Nachleben, Heft 51, Göttingen: Vandenhoeck und Ruprecht, 1978.
Siegel, Rudolph E., *Galen's System of Physiology and Medicine: An Analysis of his Doctrines and Observations on Bloodflow, Respiration, Humans and Internal Diseases*, Basel and NY: S. Karger, 1968.
Smith, Morton, *Jesus the Magician*, NY: Harper and Row, 1978.
Smith, Wesley D., *The Hippocratic Tradition*, Ithaca, NY: Cornell University Press, 1979.
Spencer, W. G., in Introduction to Vol. II of *Celsus* in Loeb Classical Library, London: W. Heinemann Ltd, 1958.
Temkin, Owsei, *Galenism: Rise and Decline of a Medical Philosophy*, Ithaca, NY: Cornell University Press, 1973.

Tiede, David L., *The Charismatic Figure as Miracle Worker*, SBLDS 1
  Missoula, Mont., 1977.
Vermes, Geza, *Jesus the Jew*, New York: Macmillan, 1973.
Wilken, Robert L., *The Christians as the Romans Saw Them*, New Haven:
  Yale University Press, 1984.

SUBJECT INDEX

AUTHOR INDEX

ANCIENT AUTHORS INDEX

INDEX OF PASSAGES QUOTED